HEALTHY VEGAN COOKING

A BEGINNER'S GUIDE TO PLANT-BASED COOKING

54 DELICIOUS VEGAN RECIPES

THOMAS CALABRIS

Check out our website at:
www.SimpleVeganDiet.com

Healthy Vegan Cooking
Publisher: Inner Vitality Systems, LLC.
Website: www.SimpleVeganDiet.com
ISBN: 978-1-951382-02-5

Copyright © 2020 by Thomas Calabris

All rights reserved. No part of this publication may be reproduced or utilized in any form or by any means, electronic or mechanical, including photocopying, recording, or by any information storage and retrieval system, without prior written permission from the publisher. All rights reserved, including the right of reproduction in whole or in part in any form. Inquiries should be addressed to the publisher.

Disclaimer

The Information presented in this publication is intended as an educational resource and is not intended as a substitute for proper medical advice. All readers are encouraged to seek proper professional and medical advice when needed.

The author and publisher of this material are not responsible in any manner whatsoever for any action or injury which may occur by reading or following the instruction in this document. The author cannot be held responsible for any personal or commercial damage caused by misinterpretation or improper use of the information.

No patent liability is assumed concerning the use of the information contained herein. Although every precaution has been taken in the preparation of this book, the publisher and author assume no responsibility for errors or omissions.

VEGAN BASED SUBSTITUTIONS FOR "NORMAL" RECIPES. 37
   Milk Substitutions 37
   Buttermilk Substitutions 37
   Butter Substitutions 37
   Egg Substitutions 38
   Cheese Substitutions 39
   Sour Cream Substitutions 39
ESSENTIAL INGREDIENTS FOR VEGAN COOKING 39
   Vegetables 39
   Fruit 40
   Grains 40
   Gluten-free 41
   Nuts and Seeds 41
   Legumes 42
ANIMAL BASED INGREDIENTS TO AVOID 42
OTHER HELPFUL FOOD TIPS 43

CHAPTER 7 – COOKING BASICS 46
HOME KITCHEN SETUP 47
BASIC COOKING TERMS 47
   ABBREVIATIONS 49
   CONVERSIONS 49

SECTION 2 – VEGAN RECIPES 52
CHAPTER 8 – CONDIMENTS 53

- Vegetable Gravy...54
- Savory Salsa Verde...55
- Pickled Jalapeño Peppers With Red Onion.................57
- Caramelized Onions...58
- Spicy Mango Salsa..60

Chapter 9 – Smoothies...........................61
- Mango Breakfast Smoothie..62
- Banana Bread and Blueberry Smoothie.....................63
- Blueberry Smoothie...64
- Spring Time Smoothie..65
- Maca Almond Smoothie...66
- Minty Avocado and Spinach Smoothie......................67
- Pumpkin and Avocado Smoothie................................68

Chapter 10 – Breakfast.........................69
- Almond Flour Pancakes..70
- Slow Cooker Apple-Cinnamon Oats............................71
- Instant Pot Steel-Cut Oats With Berries.................73
- Vegan Chickpea Omelet..75

Chapter 11 – Soups and Stock..................77
- Creamy Wild Rice and Mushroom Soup......................78
- Chilled Cucumber Avocado Soup with Fresh Dill. 80
- Creamy Broccoli Soup..81

Garlic Castilian Soup...83

Roasted Yellow Tomato Soup..................................84

Roasted Tomatoes and Fennel Soup......................86

Spicy Sweet Corn Chowder....................................88

Homemade Vegetable Stock..................................90

Chapter 12 – Salads............................92

Mixed Berry Salad with Raspberry Vinaigrette....93

Garden Salad In a Mason Jar with Balsamic Dressing... 94

Roasted Beets, Citrus, And Fennel Salad.................96

Mexican Chopped Salad with Avocado Dressing.....98

Grilled Corn And Cherry Tomato Salad................100

Chapter 13 – Side Dishes And Snacks...103

Mashed Cauliflower With Garlic and Chives.......104

Curried Cauliflower Mash......................................105

Savory Butternut Squash Noodles.........................106

Mediterranean Roasted Vegetables.......................108

Roasted Rosemary Potatoes..................................110

Tuscan Wiiite Beans with Sage..............................111

Crispy Kale Chips..114

Spicy Sweet Potato Wedges with Savory Coconut Yogurt Dip... 116

Chapter 14 – Main Dishes..................119

Spicy Peanut Rice Noodles With Broccoli & Bell Peppers.................. 120

Sweet Potato Buddha Bowl with Sriracha Hummus 121

Spicy Black Bean Taco Wraps with Guacamole....123

Veggie Burgers.. 125

Herb Roasted Veggies..................................... 127

Vegan Chili... 128

Vegan Pita Pizzas... 130

Chapter 15 – Desserts........................132

Instant Pot Blueberry Maple Compote................. 133

Chocolate Hazelnut Truffles............................. 134

Blueberry & Cashew Cheesecake...................... 136

Blueberry & Pecan Crumble............................. 138

Cinnamon & Pumpkin Fudge............................ 139

Coconut Maple Fudge..................................... 140

Coconut & Peanut Butter Balls........................ 141

Chia Raspberry Pudding.................................. 142

Pumpkin and Peanut Butter Pudding................ 143

Strawberry Banana Granola Parfaits................ 144

From The Author..............................146

REFERENCES..**147**
ABOUT THE AUTHOR................................**153**
BOOKS BY THE AUTHOR..........................**154**

Healthy Vegan Cooking

SECTION 1 – VEGAN COOKING

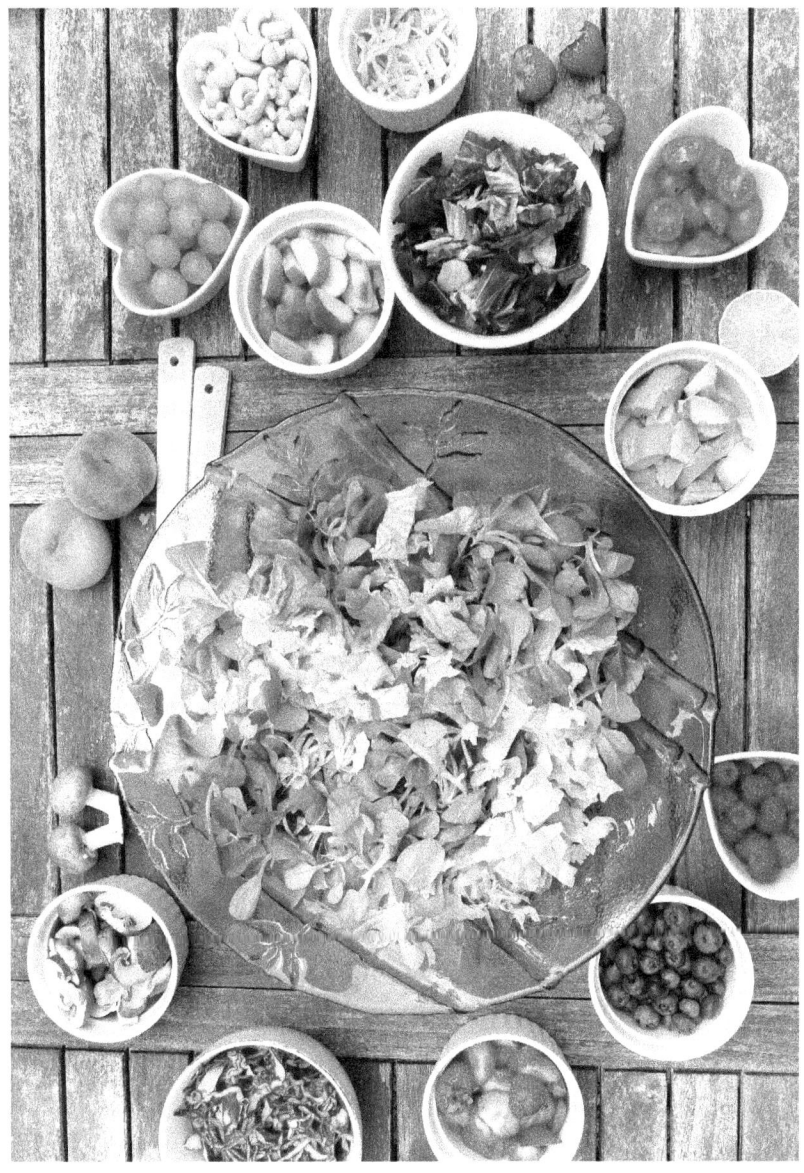

Healthy Vegan Cooking

"The love for all living creatures is the most notable attribute of man."
- Charles Darwin

"The greatness of a nation and it's moral progress can be judged by the way its animals are treated."
- Mahatma Gandhi

"Nothing will benefit human health and increase changes for survival of life on Earth as much as the evolution to a vegetarian diet."
- Albert Einstein

"I have no doubt that it is a part of the destiny of the human race, in its gradual improvement, to leave off eating animals, as surely as the savage tribes have left off eating each other when they came in contact with the more civilized."
- Henry David Thoreau

"My body will not be a tomb for other creatures."
- Leonardo da Vinci

Healthy Vegan Cooking

CHAPTER 1 – INTRODUCTION

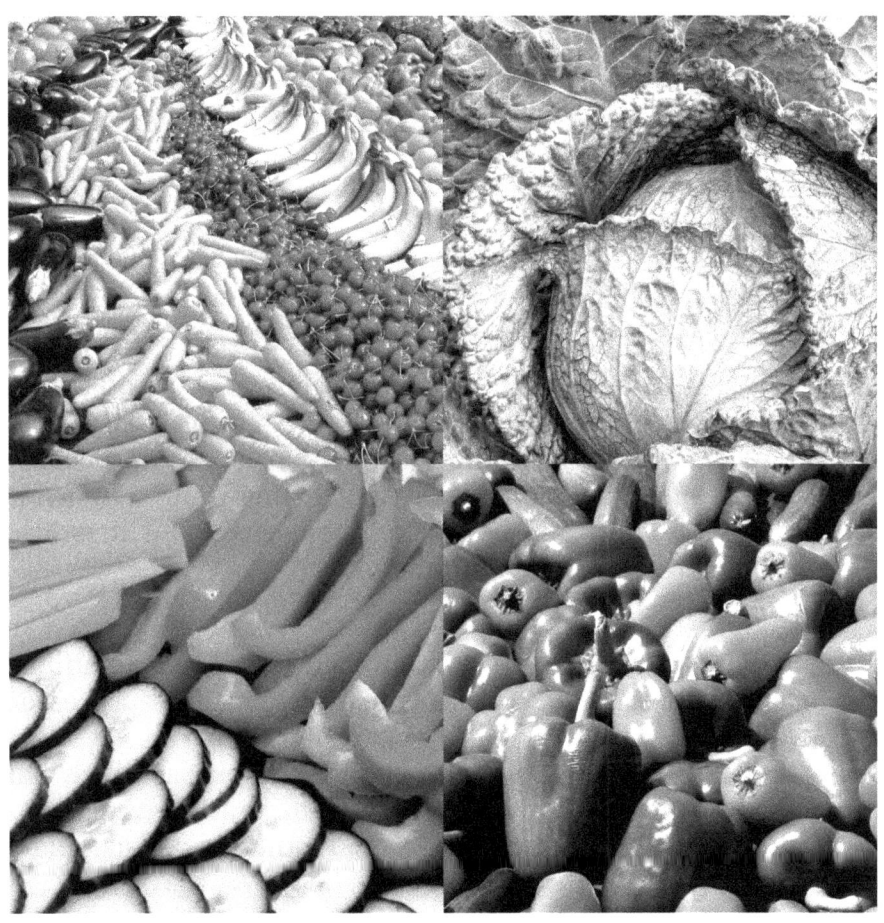

Healthy Vegan Cooking

There has been much talk about vegan diets in the last few years. If you have been wondering exactly what a vegan diet is and how to begin, then this book is for you. In this book, we will explore what veganism means and of course, how to begin a vegan diet.

Veganism refers to a way of life that excludes the use of any animal products; this means eating a vegan diet and avoiding products with animal parts, like leather and furs. However, there are different types of vegans, and not all are so strict. Some will eat a vegan diet, but still use animal products in non-dietary products. We will cover more of this later.

Veganism is a term that includes diet, ethical treatment of animals, and environmental concerns.

So why do people decide to become a vegan? Some people do it for health considerations such as to lose weight or to deal with chronic health conditions. Some people become vegan because they love animals and don't want to see them harmed. Some decide that it is not only better for themselves, but it is also cleaner and better for the environment.

A vegan diet is a healthy, plant-based diet. It excludes all animal products and derivatives. It also means eating less processed foods and processed fats. On a vegan diet, you will eat more vegetables, legumes, nuts, fruits, grains, and seeds, which has tremendous benefits. Many studies indicate that the vegan diet contains more fiber, antioxidants, and other beneficial plant compounds. [1]

A vegan diet is often richer in magnesium, folate, vitamin A, C, and E as well as potassium. However, proper planning is warranted to ensure that you get sufficient amounts of iron, calcium, zinc, iodine, vitamin B6 and B12, and essential fatty acids.

On a vegan diet, it is important to minimize "carbs" (simple carbohydrates that have little nutritional value, spike your blood sugar, and cause unwanted pounds). With the vegan diet, you will find it easy to create a meal plan that includes nutrient-dense whole food.

A vegan diet can help you to shed those unwanted pounds! Observational studies show that vegans tend to have a lower BMI and tend to be thinner. [8] Vegan diets are more effective for weight loss because of the decrease in excessive protein, natural calorie restriction, and cutting back on processed and refined foods. When eating vegan, you're more likely to feel full as well.

If you have type 2 diabetes, going vegan can help you as you may also suffer from declining kidney function. Additionally, vegans often have lower blood sugar levels and higher insulin sensitivity. They can have anywhere from a 50-78% lower risk of type 2 diabetes as well. [8] If you take medication for high blood sugar, going vegan can help to eliminate or decrease the dose that you need. By replacing meat with plant-based protein, you can reduce the risk of poor kidney function or prevent kidney disease from getting worse. [16] If you're diabetic, it can also help to relieve systemic distal polyneuropathy symptoms, which cause severe burning pain. [17]

About a third of all cancers are preventable, and one of the main factors is your diet. Eating legumes regularly can help to reduce the risk of colorectal cancer by 9-18%. [2] Eat seven portions of vegetables or fresh fruit daily can lower your risk of dying from cancer by up to 15%. [6]

Going vegan means that you'll add more vegetables, fruits, and legumes into your diet, helping you to lower the risk for both developing and dying from cancer. Vegan diets also include soy products which can help to reduce the risk of breast cancer. [18] By avoiding some animal products, you can reduce the risk of colon, prostate and breast cancer too. Without smoked or processed meats, you're less likely to be at risk of other cancers as well. [19] Also, dairy products are known to increase the risk of prostate cancer. Going vegan eliminates these from your diet.

CHAPTER 2 – VEGANISM

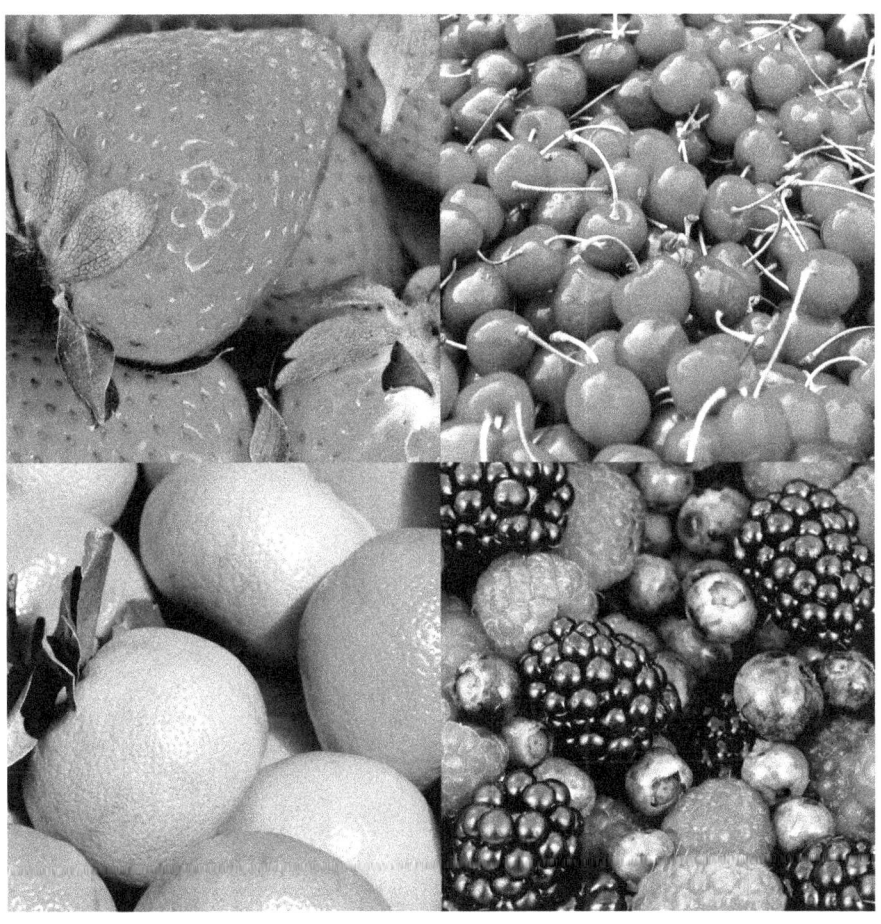

As we have mentioned previously, veganism means to eat a vegan diet and sometimes to live a vegan lifestyle. There are many different reasons for going vegan, which means there are different types of vegans. Here are some types of vegans.

Dietary Vegans

A dietary vegan is someone who does not eat any animal products; this means that you would not eat anything that contained animal by-products, including dairy, eggs, meat, and even honey. However, veganism can also extend beyond the diet and include ethical and environmental concerns as well. For the purposes of this book, we will focus on dietary veganism.

Ethical Vegans

Ethical vegans are against the use of animals for any reason whatsoever. They do not buy or use any products that are made using animals. This would include things such as fur rugs or coats, leather, soap made from tallow, cosmetics, hair care products, skincare products, and any products that are tested on animals.

Environmental vegans

Environmental vegans are similar to ethical vegans, except they do not use animal products because they believe that industrial farming is bad for the environment and is unsustainable. For example, environmental vegans think that the production of cow-derived products is harmful to the environment because the cows produce methane that contributes to greenhouse gases.

HISTORY OF VEGANISM

While the term veganism has only been around less than 100 years, history has shown evidence that some people avoided animal products over 2000 years ago. [20]

In terms of modern history, veganism is not that old of an idea; less than 100 years believe it or not. The word "vegan" was first coined by a man named Donald Watson. In November 1944, he co-founded the Vegan Society in England, which still exists today. [21]

The group who founded this society wanted to do more than only avoid eating meat. They also eliminated dairy and eggs; thus, veganism was born. Not only did the Vegan Society not eat any food made from animals, but they also explained early on that they didn't use any animal products. So from the beginning, the members of the Vegan Society viewed veganism as something more than just related to diet. [20]

Since the 1940s, veganism has increased in popularity. It's easy to see why. We live in the information era. Today, we have easy access to digital information online in the form of eBooks, audiobooks, articles, and videos. So it is no surprise that the benefits of going vegan became very popular once published.

Also, there are more restaurants offering vegan options. And, more grocery stores are offering a wider selection of vegan-friendly foods.

According to GlobalData, surveys showed that the number of Americans that called themselves vegan increased from just 1% in 2014 to 6% in 2017. [22] Thus, in 2017, over 19 million Americans called themselves vegan.

VEGANISM AND HEALTH

Veganism has been associated with good health, which is a big reason why more people are going vegan. The ethical considerations around eating other living beings are a sore point for most other vegans, but the health benefits should not be overlooked.

Studies have shown that plant-based diets not only reduce the risk of heart disease, but they also help to control type 2 diabetes and cancer. A plant-based diet can even help to prevent premature death. [8][23][24] Another common reason that people lean toward veganism is because of concerns over eating chicken, cows, and other animals that are given large amounts of antibiotics and hormones.

In the next chapter, we will discuss the basics of a vegan diet. Then in the following chapter, we will discuss the health benefits of a vegan diet in greater detail.

Chapter 3 – Vegan Diet

The vegan diet isn't just super easy to follow. It is also a great way to keep the body healthy while staying full and happy. With that said, the question arises, what exactly can you eat while on a vegan diet? And more importantly, what do you have to avoid?

What to Eat

What can you eat? Contrary to the myth that vegans can't eat anything but "grass," there is a wide range of options available to you. Besides the obvious choices such as vegetables and fruit, you can also eat nuts, seeds, tofu, legumes, and plant milk, such as coconut milk or soy. Here's a list of food items that you should stock in your kitchen.

- Vegetables
- Fruit
- Legumes
- Tofu
- Tempeh
- Seitan
- Sea salt
- Pepper
- Soy sauce
- Assorted spices and herbs
- Mustard
- Vegan mayonnaise
- Vegan butter

Healthy Vegan Cooking

- Extra virgin olive oil
- Grape seed oil
- Peanut oil
- Coconut oil
- Palm shortening
- Assorted vinegar
- Whole grains (wheat, barley, rye, rice)
- Flour (whole wheat, soy, almond, chickpea, and others)
- Whole-grain bread
- Plant-based protein powder (soy, rice, pumpkin)
- Plant-based milk (soy, almond, cashew, coconut)
- Nuts and nut butter
- Avocado and avocado oil and butter

You can also spice up your food with a combination of herbs and salt, but it is recommended to limit your sodium intake is between 1,000-1,500 mg per day. If you want to use salt, use sea salt or kosher salt that does not have added ingredients like anti-caking agents, which are not good for you.

Eat foods like olives, tofu, avocados, seeds, and nuts in moderation. No more than 15 to 20 percent of your calories should come from these sources. [3] Everyone has different preferences and needs, so experiment with different amounts to find out what suits your needs.

It is best to eat more complex carbohydrate vegetables, which contains lots of bulk and fiber. This will give you enough to eat and will give you that full feeling without stuffing yourself. Also, limit the amount of simple carbohydrates, like starches, sugars, and processed flours, which can spike your blood sugar.

It is best to limit your fruit intake and only stick to fruits that are low in simple carbohydrates and sugar. These include:

- Blackberries
- Strawberries
- Raspberries
- Blueberries

Don't be afraid to try new vegetables and cook them in different ways, especially if you are not a fan of raw food.

What NOT to Eat

From a diet perspective, vegans refrain from eating animal or animal-based foods. The list of things that you shouldn't eat in veganism is pretty simple. If it comes with an animal association, you cut it loose. That includes meat and poultry, starting with beef and chicken and everything in between. Fish-based products are also off-limits. Also, anchovies, shrimp, scallops, and crabs are all off the list. Dairy products such as milk, whey, cheese, and ice cream are also off-limits. The same goes for eggs, honey, and gelatin.

Any food containing animal fat and enzymes (chocolates, cheeses, salad dressings, sauces, and bread) should also be removed from your shopping list. Some vegans even avoid eating vegan food that is heavily processed, like flours, oils, and fake meat and dairy products.

It is also important to avoid highly processed foods that have little nutritional value but will cause you to pack on the pounds. Here's a brief list; however, there are many others.

- White pasta
- White bread
- Cereals with low fiber and added sugar

- Soda, diet soda
- Artificial sweeteners
- Fruit juices with additives and sweeteners
- Potato chips
- Crackers
- Pretzels

You can top your food with a natural sweetener, but it is recommended to limit the highly processed sweeteners.

It is best not to consume packaged vegetarian and vegan meat substitutes. The majority of them have a high amount of simple carbohydrates (we will sometimes refer to this as high-carbs) and are heavily processed. Some veggie burgers are a better option.

Genetically modified or non-fermented soy products are not healthy and should be avoided. Also, I recommend limiting or eliminating all foods that have been genetically modified (GMO). GMOs have been linked to a variety of health issues, including digestive issues, food allergies, liver problems, and more. [11]

LIFESTYLE FACTORS

Sleep

Everyone needs rest; it's an essential process that enables the body to digest, recover, and heal. Adults need at least 8 hours' sleep per day. However, those on a high-carb (that is a high amount of simple carbohydrates) diet need between 9-10 hours' sleep per day.

Hydration

It is important that you drink enough purified water to maintain good health. I don't recommend regular tap water that has many chemicals. It is best to filter or distill the water before drinking it. Adults should consume about 64 ounces, or a half-gallon, of water per day. Also, it is best to drink water throughout the day. People on a non-vegetarian diet should consume between 1 to 1½ gallons of water per day, despite consuming more water-based foods. [2] Since the non-vegetarian diet has a slight diuretic effect, they need to consume more water than usual to avoid becoming dehydrated.

Exercise

A moderate amount of exercise is recommended daily. It is best to get at least 30 minutes of physical activity each day. More activity may be needed for losing weight. Add aerobic activity and strength training for the best results. Moderate exercise is recommended to prevent overexertion, which could lead to medical issues like dehydration, injury, or extreme weight loss.

Calories

Many experts have continuously disagreed on the average recommended daily calorie intake amount. The typical amount is between 1,800–2,000 calories for women and 2,500 calories for men. The numbers are entirely different for those on a non-vegetarian diet. They require between 2,500–3,000 calories per day and may eat as much as 6,000 calories when they are very active. [8]

COMMON MYTHS ABOUT A VEGAN DIET

There are plenty of myths that surround a vegan diet, but here are a few of the most common ones.

Myth #1: You Don't Get Adequate Protein On A Vegan Diet

This is definitely the most common myth vegans will hear about their diet. People associate protein with meat. They think that the only way someone could get enough protein in their diet is by eating meat.

First, let's talk about how much protein is enough per day. The Recommended Dietary Allowance (RDA) for protein is 0.8 grams per kilogram of body weight. Thus, a person that weighs 150 pounds should eat about 54 grams of protein. [25]

There are plenty of options to get enough protein as a vegan. Here are a few. [26][27]

Healthy Vegan Cooking

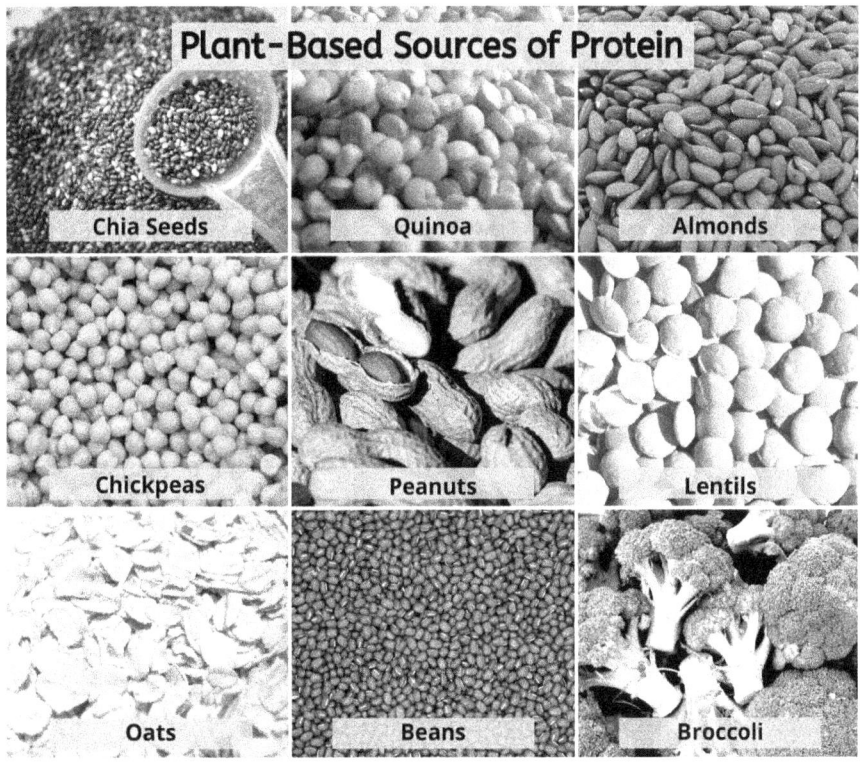

Healthy Vegan Cooking

Vegan Source	Protein (g)	Source Amount
Almonds	16.5 g	½ cup
Black Beans	14 g	1 cup
Broccoli	4 g	1 medium stalk
Buckwheat	5.5 g	1 cup
Chia Seeds	2 g	1 tablespoon
Chickpeas	11 g	1 cup
Hemp Seeds	6 g	2 tablespoons
Lentils	18 g	1 cup
Nutritional Yeast	4 g	2 tablespoons
Oats	6 g	1 cup
Peanuts	20.5 g	½ cup
Pumpkin Seeds	8 g	1.5 ounces
Russet Potato	8 g	1 large
Quinoa	8 g	1 cup
Tempeh	17 g	½ cup
Tofu	9 g	3 ounces

Myth #2: Vegan Diets Are Too Expensive

Some people think that eating healthy food, such as leafy green vegetables, is too expensive. In fact, foods like beans, fruits, vegetables, rice, and other vegan staples are not as expensive as meat. Moreover, some of these food items like rice and beans have a much longer shelf life than meat does.

Let's look at it from a different perspective. Eating meat is more costly than eating a vegan diet. First, meat is high in saturated fat, preservatives, growth hormones, and antibiotics. This is unhealthy and will cost you your health in the long run. Also, eating a vegan diet with organic vegetables, fruit, and grains, for example, is healthier and it doesn't necessarily mean more out of your pocket.

Remember, meat is very costly. It could not only cost you your health, but your medical bills will be much higher. This could also contribute to higher medical insurance. So you may be paying to ruin your health. Of course, if you must eat meat, then at least eat organic meat that doesn't have growth hormones, antibiotics, and that was raised on pesticide-free grains.

Myth #3: You Can't Get Enough Calcium On A Vegan Diet

It is important to point out that milk and cheese aren't the only sources of calcium. You can get plenty of calcium from plant-based sources, including soybeans, beans, some nuts and seeds, kale, spinach, broccoli, and figs.

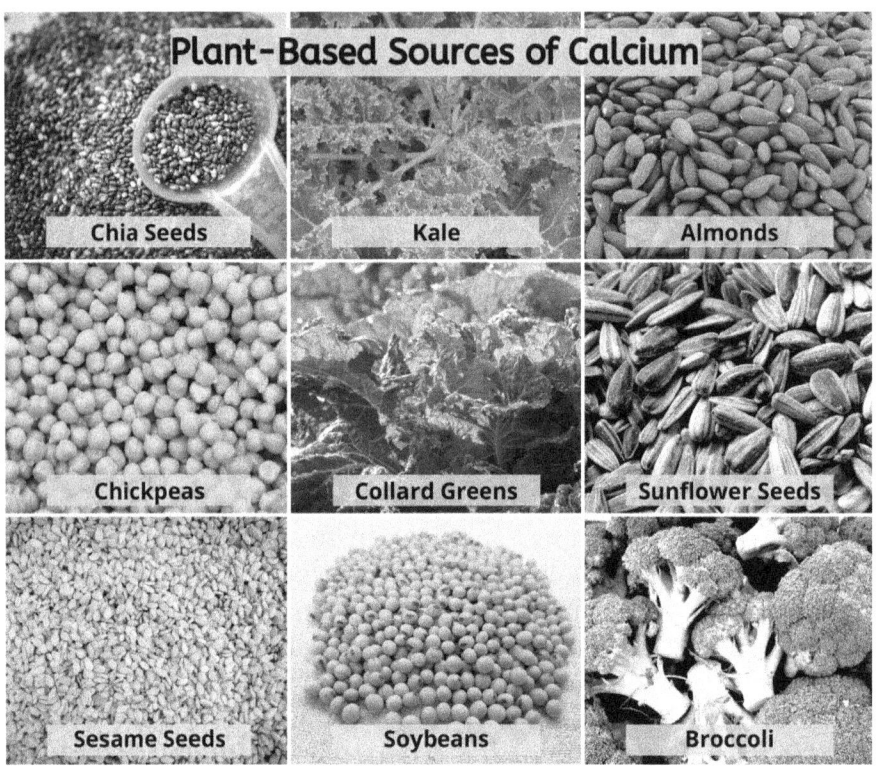

The Recommended Daily Allowance (RDA) of calcium for adults is 1,000 mg. The following table shows the vegan calcium sources, along with the source amount and with the calcium amount in milligrams. [28][29][30][31]

Healthy Vegan Cooking

Vegan Source	Calcium (mg)	Source Amount
Almonds	378 mg	1 cup
Black Beans	294 mg	1 cup
Blackstrap Molasses	100 mg	2 tablespoons
Broccoli	62 g	1 cup, cooked
Chia Seeds	179 mg	2 tablespoon
Chickpeas	80 mg	1 cup, cooked
Collard greens	268 mg	1 cup chopped/boiled
Figs	18 mg	1 raw fig
Kale (raw)	101 mg	1 cup
Navy Beans	126 mg	1 cup, cooked
Orange	50 mg	1 orange
Pinto Beans	79 mg	1 cup, cooked
Sesame Seeds	88 mg	1 tablespoon
Soybeans	175 mg	1 cup, cooked
Sunflower Seed Kernels	109 mg	1 cup
Tahini	128 mg	2 tablespoons
Tempeh	184 mg	1 cup
Tofu	870 mg	1 cup
Turnip Greens	197 mg	1 cup, cooked

Myth #4: You Need to Eat Meat to Be Healthy

Many factors contribute to being healthy. While meat may provide protein, calcium, and iron, it doesn't provide much in the way of antioxidants, phytonutrients, or fiber. Meat is also a source of cholesterol and saturated fat, which are contributors to cardiovascular disease, and it has been associated with gastrointestinal issues. Research has also shown that eating a vegan diet can reduce your risk of heart disease and type 2 diabetes. A vegan diet can also lower cholesterol and blood pressure. [3] And as we have seen, you can get enough protein and calcium. Chapter 4 of this book goes into much greater detail on the health benefits of a vegan diet.

Myth #5: You'll Be Hungry a Lot

This idea comes from people who eat meat and think that's the only way you can have a filling and satisfying meal. How could you possibly get full eating vegetables? Well, it's quite easy! Many foods you'll eat on a vegan diet are rich in fiber, which will help to keep you full longer. Beans and leafy green vegetables are rich in fiber, making it hard not to get and stay full!

CHAPTER 4 – HEALTH BENEFITS OF A VEGAN DIET

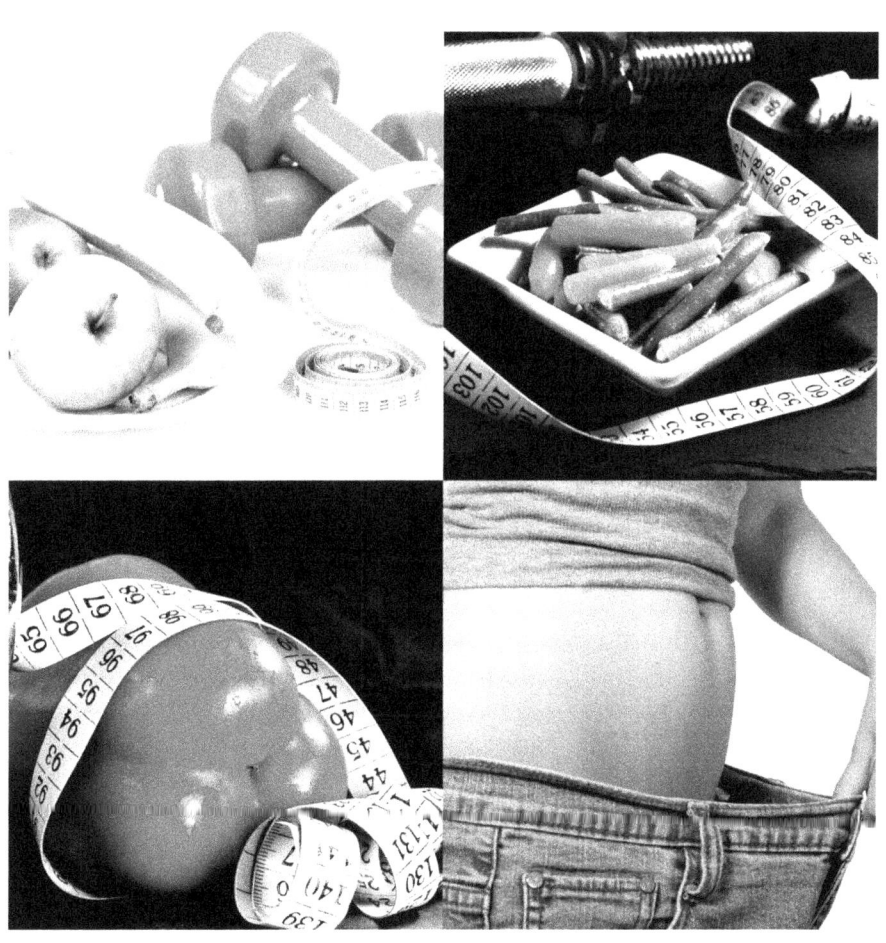

There are many health benefits that a vegan diet will provide to you. The standard American Diet (SAD) today isn't a very good one. Many people eat fast food daily, and they eat way too many unhealthy fats and simple sugars.

It's more convenient to drive through and get fast food after a long day at work instead of preparing a healthy meal. However, poor eating choices have consequences. Heart disease causes about 610,000 American deaths each year. Most of these deaths could have been prevented with a proper diet and exercise routine. [1]

Also, there are many restaurants you won't be able to eat at. And, you'll have to plan ahead for parties and other events that likely won't have vegan-friendly options. With all that said, you must remember why you started a vegan diet in the first place. Yes, going on a vegan diet isn't going to be the easiest thing in the world to do, but the gained health benefits are worth it. The following benefits are some of the common reasons why people start a vegan diet in the first place.

GOOD FOR THE ENVIRONMENT

When many people think about going green or saving the planet, they typically think about recycling more or reducing the use of plastic. That's a great start, but becoming a vegan can do more than you might think. For example, the livestock segment is the biggest producer of nitrous oxide and methane gases. Many people think that carbon dioxide is the worst gas that contributes the most to climate change, but it's actually methane and nitrous oxide.

While carbon dioxide may not be the most damaging gas for climate change, it still has an impact. Approximately 9% of carbon dioxide emission in the United States comes from the livestock segment. [10]

Thus, going vegan will help to reduce the amount of methane, nitrous oxide, and carbon dioxide released into the atmosphere since vegans don't eat animals.

Another factor that is often overlooked when it comes to livestock and the environment is deforestation. Animals are herded together and kept in one place, which requires large amounts of land for them to live on. As a result, the destruction of forests can trigger climate change and destroy natural habitats for animals native to the forests.

KIND REGARDS FOR ANIMALS

Ethical vegans feel that the harming and killing of animals for any purpose is wrong. They believe that animals should have rights, like humans.

Many people are unaware of what it feels like to kill animals for their food. They would likely feel bad if they watched the slaughter of an animal.

By going on a vegan diet, you can help save animals everywhere. According to PETA, a vegan saves almost 200 animals per year. [32]

To further illustrate this point, let's take a look at some statistics. The number of pounds of meat produced for August in 2017 [9]:

- Commercial Red Meat Production: 4.63 billion pounds
- Beef Production: 2.4 billion pounds
- Veal Production: 6.4 million pounds
- Pork Production: 2.21 billion pounds
- Lamb and Mutton Production: 12.8 million pounds

As you can see, these meat production numbers are high. You might be thinking to yourself, "How can one person going vegan make a difference?" Well, that's similar to the reasoning of, "Why should I vote? My vote won't change the results of the election?" Imagine if everyone thought like that though. What if people didn't vote because they believed that their single vote didn't matter? Then any single person's vote would matter a lot!

Ultimately, it's not about the single vote or a single person going vegan. It's about the principle behind it. It's about standing up for what you believe in and focusing on what you're in control of. While you can't make everyone become a vegan, you can be a good living example of a vegan for the people that are around you.

They'll see how much you care, and they'll be able to tell how passionate you are about animals. They might get curious and ask questions. Or they may even become vegan themselves one day. You'll never know unless you try!

IMPROVE YOUR HEALTH

One of the main reasons that people become vegan is for the amazing health benefits. People who follow a vegan diet have a lower risk for the following diseases [7]:

- Decreased risk for heart disease by 26-68%
- Decreased risk for prostate cancer by 35%
- Decreased risk for type 2 diabetes by 25-49%
- Decreased risk for hypertension by 55%

These numbers show how much of a positive impact eating a vegan diet can have on a person's health considering that approximately 1 in 4 males and 1 in 5 females die from cancer in the U.S. Also, about 1 in 3 Americans have high blood pressure. [6]

Here are some other benefits you'll likely experience by starting a vegan diet.

Weight Loss

Studies have shown that people on a plant-based diet can lose more weight than those not on a plant-based diet. [1] This results from consuming more natural and unprocessed foods. These foods provide you with healthy nutrients, and they contain fewer calories than the processed foods that people tend to eat.

Thus, the foods on a vegan diet are nutrient-dense and have a low caloric density. Nutrient density refers to the amount of beneficial nutrients that are in food relative to its weight. Caloric density refers to the number of calories that are in food relative to its weight.

Processed foods have a low nutrient density and a high caloric density. This means that while they have a high number of calories, they won't keep you satiated for very long since they are low in nutrition that the body needs.

Imagine eating 100 calories of vegetables versus eating 100 calories of candy. You would have to eat a lot more of the vegetables to reach that 100-calorie mark than you would eat the candy. Moreover, the vegetables provide your body with beneficial vitamins, minerals, antioxidants, phytonutrients, and fiber. But, the candy will only give you a sugar rush. Finally, you won't be hungry soon after eating the vegetables, but the candy will do little to fill you up.

This is something very important to think about. It's not just the excess calories in junk food that causes you harm. It's also the lack of fiber and nutrients, among other things. This will cause you to go back and eat more soon after your meal, simply because it didn't meet your body's nutritional demands.

Improve Digestive Health

Some fruits and vegetables contain a good amount of prebiotics and probiotics. Prebiotics are non-digestible carbohydrates that perform as fuel for probiotics. Prebiotics act in a symbiotic relationship when combined with probiotics.

Probiotics are a type of beneficial bacteria that live in different organs, and their main function is to help aid in digestion. Probiotics also help control bad bacteria and fungi. When probiotics are low, the bad bacteria or fungi can grow and infect the organ and even the entire body. When the bad bacteria grow out of control, they also consume the nutrients that were meant for the body thus robbing you of key nutrients and possibly causing nutritional deficiencies. [33][34]

Of course, it's great to consume more of the healthy nutrients that our bodies need. However, it's not how many nutrients you eat that matters. It is how many nutrients your body digests and absorbs that makes the difference. Thus, you can consume all the healthy foods you want, but your body must be able to properly digest, absorb, and use the nutrition from the food.

This is why it's critical to consume more foods that contain large amounts of prebiotics and probiotics. Here's a list of a few things you can eat on a vegan diet that contains a healthy amount of either prebiotics or probiotics:

- Fermented vegetables, like kimchi or sauerkraut
- Kombucha
- Apple cider vinegar
- Coconut kefir
- Olives
- Miso
- Tempeh

Consume more of these foods to supply your digestive tract with more healthy bacteria. This will aid in the absorption of key nutrients from the other foods you consume.

Enzymes and Antioxidants

When you want to get and stay healthy, eating wholesome foods is a great start, but it's not everything. You need a complete defense to help protect you from disease as much as possible.

This is where enzymes and antioxidants can come into play. Being on a vegan diet will allow you to consume more fresh fruits and vegetables. And if you're consuming a lot of this produce raw, you can consume even more antioxidants and enzymes.

Enzymes are a substance that acts as a catalyst to bring about a biochemical reaction. Thus, enzymes enable your body to break down food particles into usable nutrients. Therefore, the more usable enzymes a food contains, the easier it will be to digest and process. Since the cooking process destroys many enzymes in food, it is essential to eat your produce raw when possible. [35]

Antioxidants remove potentially damaging oxidizing agents, free radicals, in a living organism. In other words, we need antioxidants to help prevent cell damage caused by oxidants. [36]

Here's a list of some foods that contain a good number of antioxidants:
- Beets
- Blueberries
- Cranberries
- Goji berries
- Kale
- Kidney beans
- Kiwis
- Pecans
- Pumpkin
- Spinach
- Strawberries

Eating more foods like these will help to prevent disease and help combat free radicals in the body.

Prevention of Syndrome X

Syndrome X is commonly referred to as metabolic syndrome. Approximately 47 million Americans have it. That's a staggering 1 out of every 6 Americans! Syndrome X itself isn't a disease. It is a collection of risk factors that increase the likelihood of getting heart disease, stroke, and diabetes. [1]

Here are the factors:
- Blood sugar: 100 mg/dL or higher
- Blood pressure: 135/85 mm Hg or higher
- Big Waistline: Over 40 inches for men and 35 inches for women
- High Amounts of Bad Cholesterol: 150 mg/dL or higher
- Low Amounts of Good Cholesterol: Less than 40 mg/dL for men and less than 50 mg/dL for women

A person with 3 or more of these risk factors may be diagnosed with Syndrome X. Eating wholesome food, like that of a vegan diet, can help to reduce the risks of developing these harmful diseases associated with metabolic syndrome.

Helps with Osteoporosis and Arthritis

Osteoporosis is a disease characterized by weak bones due to low bone density. Anyone can develop osteoporosis, though, women are more than four times more likely to develop osteoporosis than men. [5] This occurs when the ovaries stop producing a key hormone, called oestrogen, once a woman goes through menopause.

At first glance, though, it wouldn't appear that a vegan diet would be good for osteoporosis. When you think of strong bones, you usually think about calcium. In a typical American diet, people get most of their calcium from sources like cheese and milk. You can't eat those foods on a vegan diet, which is why most people would think that a vegan diet is bad for osteoporosis.

However, there are plenty of vegan-friendly foods that are high in calcium, including:
- Kale
- Spinach
- Figs
- Turnip Greens
- Black-Eyed Peas
- Almond Milk

Another misconception about bone health is that only calcium matters. Other vitamins and minerals are necessary for strong bones such as vitamins D and K, magnesium, and potassium. Eating beans, leafy greens, and getting some sunlight will provide you with these key nutrients.

Arthritis is inflammation of the joints that cause pain and stiffness and can worsen with age. Research has shown that a probiotic-rich vegan diet can help reduce the symptoms of arthritis, such as pain, morning stiffness, and joint swelling. Whereas, people on an omnivorous diet did not see these benefits. [5]

Chapter 5 – Top Five Types Of The Vegan Diet

Now, believe it or not, veganism is a pretty popular topic, and as such, there are quite a few types of veganism. However, they all fit into five basic types.

Dietary Veganism

Dietary vegans eat a plant-based diet and avoid any form of animal-based food products. That is, they do not eat anything that at any point was part of an animal. They often choose a vegan diet as means to deal with health issues or to lose weight.

However, they do use animal-based products that aren't food-related. For example, they may use animal products in their makeup or as part of their clothes, such as wool or fur.

Whole-food Veganism

A whole-food vegan only eats foods that are rich in "whole" foods such as fruits, veggies, whole grains, nuts, and seeds. Thus, they choose to exclude processed and junk food, even if they are free of any form of animal product. This is sometimes referred to as "clean eating." [39]

Junk Food Veganism

A junk-food vegan is the exact opposite of the whole-food vegan. They eat lots of various types of processed and synthetic foods. Their only concern is that their food is free of animal products. Some individuals who are new to the vegan diet will load up on substitutions, like fake cheese or fake meat, instead of going for healthier options like nut butter or tofu.

Raw Food Veganism

The raw-food vegan is the sushi samurai of the vegan community. These vegans eat mostly raw foods such as fruits, vegetables, nuts, and seeds. Even when they do cook them, they make a point not to cook them over 115 degrees Fahrenheit. People are often attracted to this type of veganism for health benefits and believe that cooking food above this temperature will result in the loss of some of its nutritional potency. [40]

Low-fat, Raw-food Veganism

And finally, we have the low-fat, raw-food vegans. These vegans, who are also known as fruitarians, are a subset of raw vegans and limit high-fat foods such as avocados or nuts. As a result, these vegans tend to almost exclusively eat fruits and a smaller group of vegetables. [37]

Weight Loss and Veganism

All altruistic issues aside, however, veganism has become part of the mainstream culture for losing weight. Compared to similar diets such as Paleo or Atkins, vegan diets have proven track records for allowing the dieter to lose weight without leaving them feeling starved. A large part of this is because of the higher dietary fiber intake of vegans, which results from their high vegetable intake. This means that even if vegans are eating larger portions, their calories are not as high as the fiber content!

Chapter 6 – Vegan Cooking Ingredients

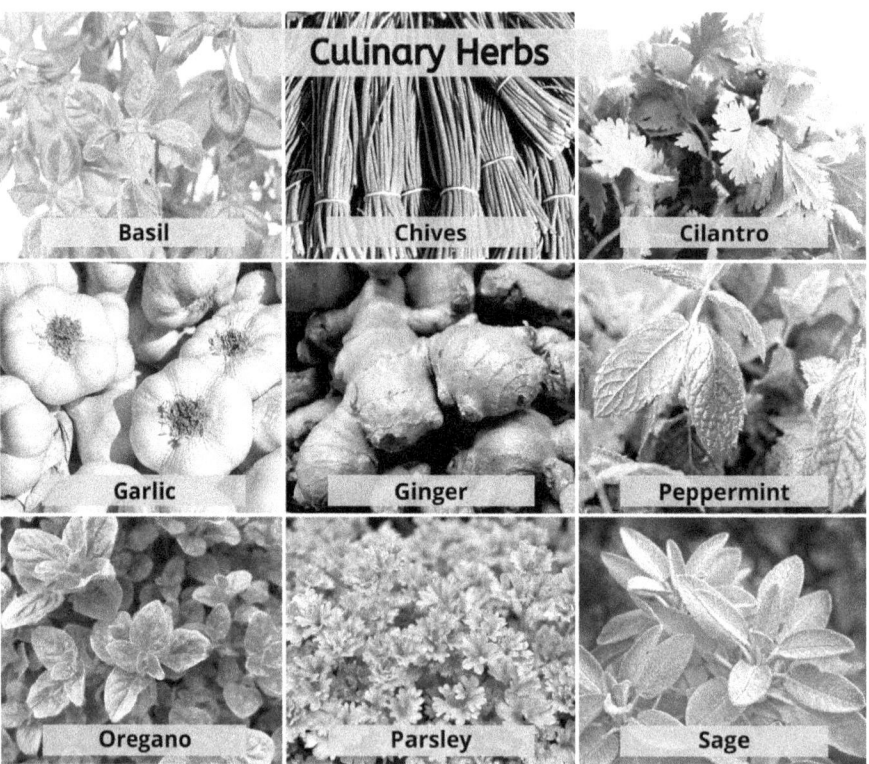

When you eliminate animal-based products from your diet, your recipes need to be updated to include vegan substitutions.

Vegan Based Substitutions for "Normal" Recipes

Some of the ingredients in the non-vegan, or "avoid at all costs" list, are typical in most recipes. So we thought you might like to have some vegan substitutions to use for normal recipes. So let's get started.

Milk Substitutions

There are a lot of plant-based milk options these days. Vegan milk includes soy, nut (almond, cashew, hazelnut, and coconut), oat, and rice milk. You can find some, if not all these at your local grocery store. You can replace 1 cup of milk with 1 cup of the plant-based milk. Be aware that not all plant-based types of milk are created equal. Steer clear of those loaded with sugars, artificial flavors, and unhealthy additives such as carrageenan, xanthan gum, and guar gum (there may be others so make sure you read the labels). And keep in mind that some plant-based types of milk are better for some recipes than others. You should test them in your recipes before your big party to make sure that it tastes best with the other ingredients.

Buttermilk Substitutions

You can make your own vegan-friendly buttermilk substitute by mixing 1 cup of vegan milk (see Milk substitutions) and one tablespoon of lemon juice or vinegar.

Butter Substitutions

Oils are great substitutes for butter, though not all options are suitable for cooking at medium to high temperatures. So, look at their cooking temperatures before using them. Good oils for high temperature cooking are sunflower oil, avocado oil, and coconut oil. Oils for medium to low-temperature cooking include regular olive oil and sesame oil. Extra virgin olive oil, flax oil, and pumpkin oil are best for salad dressings or unheated foods.

Egg Substitutions

Eggs are typically used in cooking/baking to bind the ingredients together. So don't worry, there are many options for egg alternatives in vegan cooking. Not all options are good for all recipes, so you may need to experiment to get the best tasting results. Here are a few options:

Applesauce is a great substitute for eggs in baking, such as muffins, cookies, and cakes. Use one-quarter of a cup of applesauce as a substitute for one egg. Unsweetened applesauce is the best. But if you use sweetened applesauce, just reduce the amount of other sweeteners in the recipe.

Bananas that are mashed or pureed are a great option for replacing eggs in some baked goods, though it likely won't work for savory dishes. Just replace 1 egg with one-half of a medium-sized banana.

Tofu can sometimes be used as an egg substitution. Put tofu in a blender and blend it until it is smooth. Then use one-quarter of a cup of smooth tofu as a substitute for one large egg.

Flour may also be used for some egg substitutions. You can use one tablespoon of flour (wheat, soy, or oat) and one tablespoon of water as a replacement for one egg. Another option is to combine one tablespoon of flour, one tablespoon of baking powder (aluminum-free) with two tablespoons of water. This mixture is a substitute for one egg.

Cheese Substitutions

Cheese substitutions are plentiful these days. There are a lot of vegan cheeses that you can find in your grocery or health food store. Vegan cheeses include cashew nut cheese, almond cheese, and Daiya brand cheese. A good alternative to Parmesan cheese is Nutritional yeast. Also, cottage cheese can be replaced with crumbled firm tofu or vegan yogurt for some recipes. Though it may not taste as good as a standalone cottage cheese side dish.

Sour Cream Substitutions

You can make a vegan-friendly version of sour cream by mixing three-quarters of a cup of coconut milk with a tablespoon of lemon juice or vinegar, either of which will give it that sour taste.

Essential Ingredients for Vegan Cooking

We have seen how simple substitutions can help convert "normal" recipes into ones that vegans can eat. Now let's go over additional ingredients that are common in the typical vegan kitchen. You will want to stock your pantry and refrigerator with these foods.

Vegetables

For a vegan diet, vegetables are the "main-dish," and so it is important to buy them as fresh as possible. Organic vegetables are best since they will not have the pesticides as their non-organic counterparts. It will be cheaper to buy vegetables that are in season and local when possible. Vegetables are great sources for fiber, phytonutrients, vitamins, and minerals.

Fruit

Fruits are loaded with antioxidants, enzymes, vitamins, and minerals. They are important for a balanced vegan diet. But, the more starchy fruit should be limited because they contain more calories. It is best to eat a variety of fruit of varying colors to maximize the amount of phytonutrients that are consumed.

Grains

Grains are another necessity when eating a vegan diet. Whole grains are best. Many products have heavily processed grains, like pasta, cookies, and cakes. They have very little nutritional value. So it is best to limit or eliminate processed grains. Instead, eat unprocessed whole grains. Unprocessed grains have more nutritional value and will have more fiber. You can use whole grains to make the unhealthy foods that you love healthier. You can even make your own flour using a high powered blender, like a Vitamix.

Here's a list of whole grains to consider:
- Wheat
- Rye
- Barley
- Brown Rice
- Spelt
- Quinoa
- Milet
- Oats
- Buckwheat

Gluten-free

If you need a gluten-free diet, then avoid all grains containing gluten, including wheat, spelt, rye, and barley. Also, if you want to eat oats, then buy gluten-free oats. While oats don't naturally have gluten, they are often crossed contaminated because they are processed on machinery that also processes wheat.

Nuts and Seeds

Nuts and seeds are not only a great source of vitamins and minerals, but they are also a great source of healthy fatty acids and protein. They are a great option for snacking on the go. You can also sprinkle them on salads and use them in baked goods. Be creative and enjoy them.

Here are some nuts to try:
- Walnuts
- Almonds
- Pecans
- Hazelnuts
- Brazil nuts
- Cashews

Here are some seeds to try:
- Flax seeds
- Hemp seeds
- Pumpkin seeds
- Sesame seeds
- Sunflower seeds

Legumes

Legumes are a great source of fiber, protein, and some vitamins, like B vitamins. Combined with other partial protein sources, like brown rice, they make a complete protein. Complete protein with all 9 essential amino acids is essential for a healthy vegan diet. They are great in soups, chili, and many other delicious dishes.

Here are some legumes to try:
- Black beans
- Black-Eyed peas
- Chickpeas (garbanzo beans)
- Kidney beans
- Cannelloni beans
- Northern beans
- Lentils
- Split peas
- Soybeans
- Pinto beans
- Peanuts

ANIMAL BASED INGREDIENTS TO AVOID

It is often difficult to determine if ingredients on a package are from animal products. So here's a list that you should avoid.

Gelatin – is derived from skin, tendons, ligaments, and bones of cows and pigs. And can be found in jellies, desserts, and supplement capsules. [12]

Casein – is a protein found in cow's milk, cheese, and other dairy products.

Albumin – is a protein from egg whites.

Milk derived products – include whey, lactase, lactose, and of course, milk from animals.

Bee derived products – include bee pollen, honey, royal jelly, and propolis.

Lard – fat from a pig.

Carmine – a red dye that is made from beetles.

Suet – fat from cows.

Tallow – a product made from suet.

This is not an exhaustive list, so check any ingredients that you don't recognize. Look it up before you buy it. You will likely be able to find a suitable alternative.

OTHER HELPFUL FOOD TIPS

Here are some other helpful food tips.

Oats – Oats are a wonderful add-on to any vegan diet. They are lower in carbohydrates than rice and act as binders for items such as burger patties, oatmeal bars, and even cookies!

Beans and Lentils – Beans and lentils are great foods that you are going to want to invest in regularly. Not only are they both great for salads and stews, but they also happen to work well in pasta dishes.

Flaxseed – Vegans run the risk of not getting enough of certain nutrition if they are not vigilant. Eating vegan doesn't always mean getting enough protein, vitamins, and minerals. Flaxseeds are a great plant-based source of protein. They are a great way to replace eggs as a source of protein. Also, they can be easily added to salads and smoothies to up the nutrition count.

Cashew Nuts – Cashews are not only great tasting, but they are also a good source for vegan milk and cheeses. Thus, they can add flavor and nutrition to your morning oatmeal or your afternoon stew.

Bananas – When it comes to fruits, bananas are the holy grail of vegans. They are super easy to eat and carry into work. Banana makes a great base, which is why they are used in oatmeal bowls, smoothies, and ice cream. Also, they are sometimes used as an egg or sugar substitute for baked goods.

Apple Cider Vinegar – Another thing that many vegans love is apple cider vinegar. If you follow the latest diet trends, you may have heard about turmeric tea with lemon and apple cider dominating the health-headlines. The product is a magic "cure." It plays a major role in weight loss and fat burning. It contains bacterial that is beneficial to the digestive tract. It is also great tasting on salads and in soups.

Lemons – As the saying goes, "When life gives you lemons, you make lemonade." But as a vegan, you can make so much more! Lemons are a great flavor enhancer in the vegan cooking arsenal. They can be used in flavored drinks, salads, rice bowls, and veggie sautés.

Dates – Dates are also an absolute wonder. Dates are a good sugar replacement for a vegan diet. They work not only in smoothies and energy balls but also in most desserts!

Frozen Berries – And finally, berries. Fresh berries are good when in season and if you eat them right away. Frozen berries will not spoil and ruin your budget and your mood. They can be taken out and dropped in your oatmeal or your muffin batter at any time. Frozen berries are the perfect sweet treat to keep you happy while you stay healthy!

Chapter 7 – Cooking Basics

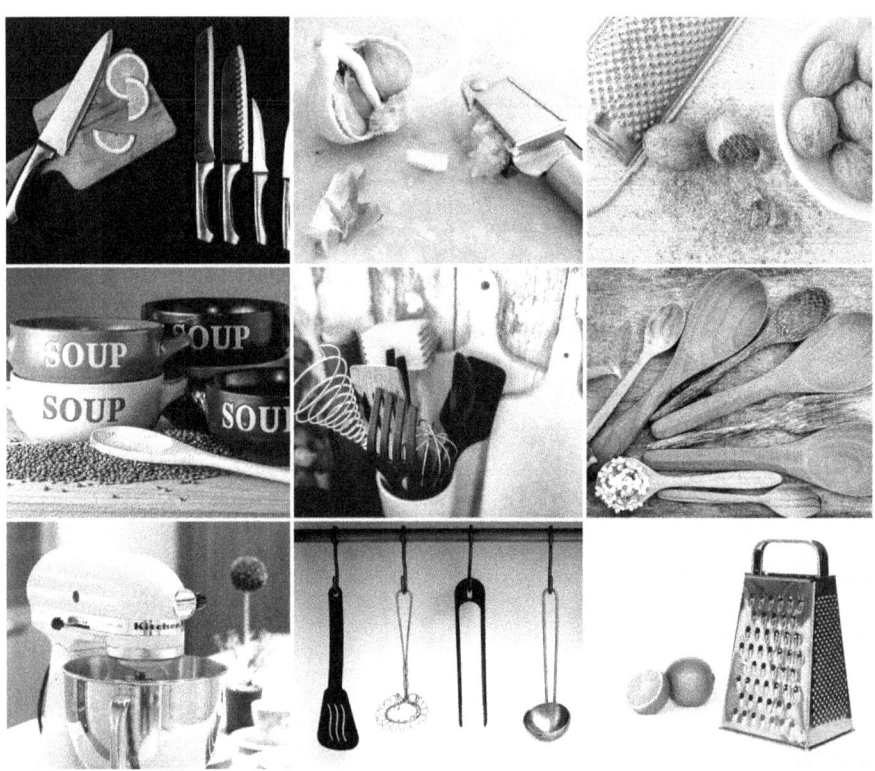

This chapter will help those that are beginning to learn how to cook. It will cover kitchen setup and basic cooking terminology. So let's get started.

Healthy Vegan Cooking

HOME KITCHEN SETUP

Your kitchen should have the necessary appliances and utensils to save you time and make cooking easier. These include:
- Electric mixer
- Blender
- Food processor
- Toaster oven
- Variety of bowls, pans, pots, and bakeware
- Utensils including spatulas, whisk, spoons, tongs, grater, peeler
- Garlic press
- Measuring spoons and cups (for dry and liquid)
- Slow Cooker
- Pressure Cooker
- Sharp knives and several cutting boards in different sizes

BASIC COOKING TERMS

Boil – Set the stove burner to a high temperature and heat a liquid or mixture to the temperature that causes it to bubble.

Simmer – Set the stove burner on low heat and heat the liquid or mixture below the boiling temperature.

Sauté cook food in a small amount of fat/oil at high temperature in a pan until done.

Frying – Heat fat/oil to a high temperature; enough to completely cover the food. Cook food in the hot fat/oil until done.

Bake – Preheat your oven to the prescribed temperature, which is typically medium to low heat (up to 375° F). Place food in the appropriate baking container (pan, casserole dish, and others) and cook for the time specified in the recipe. Food may be covered or uncovered.

Roast – Preheat your oven to a higher temperature (like 400 degrees F or above). Food is typically cooked uncovered until done.

Broil – Set the oven on broil mode. Place the food on a pan, uncovered, and put into the oven. The food is directly exposed to the high heat and is cooked one side at a time.

Mash – Place the food in a bowl and crush or smash the food to a softer, smooth texture.

Whip – Place the ingredient to be whipped into a bowl. Beat the ingredient, which adds air to make air pockets, and it becomes "fluffy," like whipping cream.

Blend – Place the ingredients in a container and mix with a spoon, whisk, blender, mixer, or food processor.

Puree – Place the cooked food, vegetables, fruit, or others, into a blender or food processor and run until it has the consistency of a smooth paste or liquid.

Grate – Rub the vegetables or other food across the grater, which makes small pieces.

ABBREVIATIONS

° = degrees
C = Centigrade (Celsius)
C,c = cup
cm = centimeter
fl oz = fluid ounce (volume)
F = Fahrenheit
g = gram
in = inch
kg = kilograms
lb = pound
ml, mL = milliliter
mg = milligrams
oz = ounce (weight)
pt = pint
qt = quart
t, tsp = teaspoon
T, tbsp, tbs = tablespoon

CONVERSIONS

Volume
1 tsp = 5 ml
1 tbsp = 15 ml
2 tbsp = 30 ml or 1 fl oz
1 cup = 240 ml or 8 fl oz
1 pt = 480 ml or 16 fl oz
2 pt = 1 qt or 32 fl oz

1 qt = 960 ml or 32 fl oz
4 qt = 1 gallon
4 tbsp = ¼ cup

Weight
1 oz = 28 g
1 lb = 454 g
2.2 lb = 1 kg

Length
1 inch = 2.54 centimeters

Temperature
32 °F = 0 °C (water freezing point)
212 °F = 100 °C (water boiling point)

°F to °C Conversion formula
°C = 5/9(°F - 32)
Example: 400 °F is approximately 204 °C

Healthy Vegan Cooking

"Let food be thy medicine, and medicine be thy food."
- Hippocrates

"The Doctor of the future will give no medicine, but will involve the patient in the proper use of food, fresh air, and exercise."
- Thomas Edison

"Whenever you find yourself on the side of the majority, it's time to pause and reflect."
- Mark Twain

"To become vegetarian is to step into the stream which leads to nirvana."
- Buddha

"I am in favor of animal rights as well as human rights. That is the way of the whole human being."
- Abraham Lincoln

"Now I can look at you in peace; I don't eat you anymore."
- Franz Kafka

SECTION 2 – VEGAN RECIPES

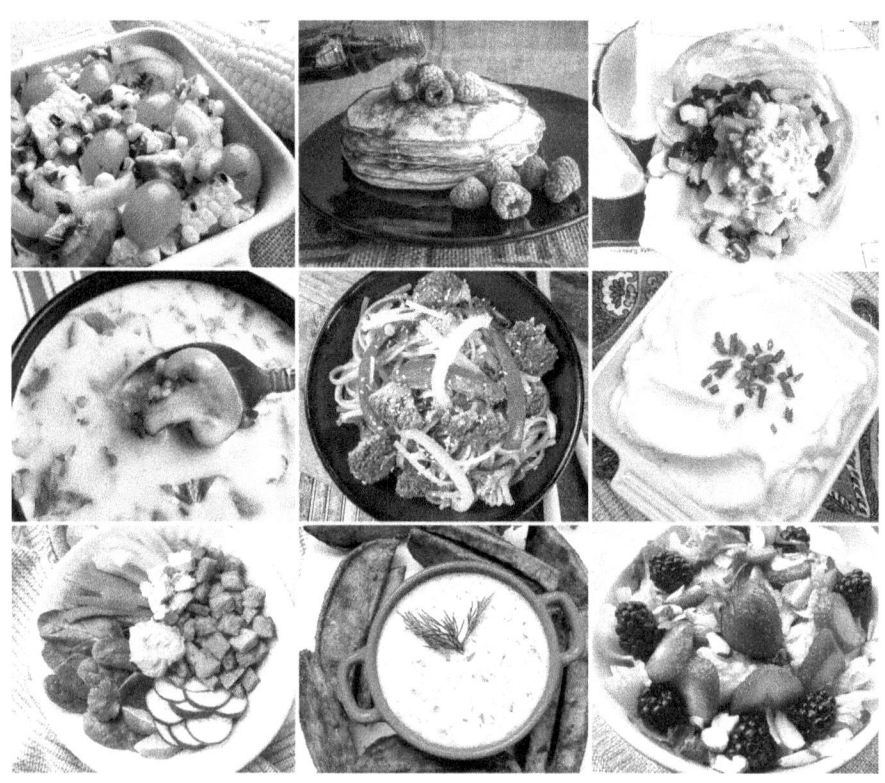

Healthy Vegan Cooking

CHAPTER 8 – CONDIMENTS

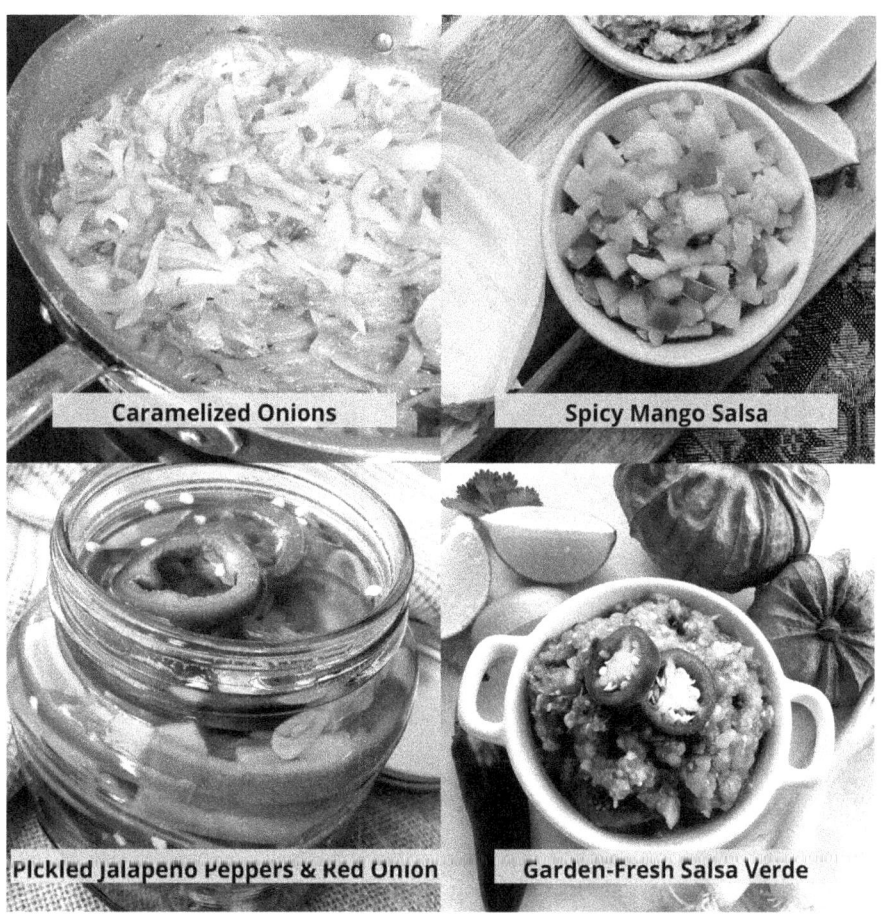

VEGETABLE GRAVY

Prep Time: 10 min
Cook Time: 12-15 min
Servings: 6

Ingredients
1 teaspoon salt
4 tomatoes, cubed
1 teaspoon chili powder
1 teaspoon coconut oil
2 onions, chopped
2 cups cubed carrots
Garnish – scallion onions, chopped

Paste Ingredients
3 garlic cloves, minced
1-inch ginger root, minced
2 teaspoons coriander powder
1 teaspoon cumin powder
Salt
Water

Directions
1. Prepare the paste by adding the paste ingredients to a food processor and blending. Add just enough water to make a paste. Set aside.
2. In a skillet, heat the oil over medium heat. Add the onions and sauté for 3-4 minutes. Then add the paste, tomatoes, and carrots, and stir fry for 6-7 minutes.
3. Garnish with scallions, and serve with rice, vegan bread, or noodles.

Nutrition Information Per Serving*

Calories: 57
Protein: 1.8 g
Carbohydrates: 11.3 g
Dietary Fiber: 2.9 g
Total Sugars: 5.5 g
Fat: 1.2 g (0.7 g saturated)

* Nutritional information is provided for educational purposes only. [13]

SAVORY SALSA VERDE

This salsa can be used in just about any recipe that calls for traditional tomato salsa. Serve with tortilla chips or add it to your favorite soup and chili recipes for extra flavor.

Prep time: 20 minutes
Cook time: 15-20 minutes
Serves: 4-6

Ingredients

1 pound Tomatillos
2 medium jalapeño peppers
3-4 cloves fresh garlic, peeled
2 tablespoons extra virgin olive oil
4 green onions, chopped
¼ cup fresh cilantro leaves
¼ cup fresh lime juice
2 teaspoons ground cumin
2 teaspoons dried oregano
Optional: 1 tablespoon maple syrup
Sea salt and black pepper

Directions

1. Preheat oven to 400 °F and line a rimmed baking sheet with parchment paper. Set aside.
2. Husk the tomatillos and cut them in half. Place the tomatillos in a single layer on a baking sheet along with whole jalapeño peppers and garlic cloves. Add a small amount of olive oil and mix gently to coat.
3. Place the baking sheet in preheated oven and roast for 15-20 minutes or until vegetables are tender. Remove from the oven and let cool for several minutes.
4. Once cool enough to handle, cut the jalapeño peppers in half and remove seeds. Then transfer the roasted veggies to a blender or food processor. Add cilantro, green onion, ground cumin, oregano, and lime juice. Pulse until ingredients are mixed, but still a little chunky.
5. Taste and add a drizzle of maple syrup to sweeten, if desired. Season with salt and black pepper. Serve immediately. You can also freeze it for later. Enjoy!

Nutrition Information Per Serving*

Calories: 86

Protein: 1.3 g

Carbohydrates: 9.8 g

Dietary Fiber: 2.1 g

Total Sugars: 5.6 g

Fat: 5.5 g (0.8 g saturated)

* Nutritional information is provided for educational purposes only. [13]

Pickled Jalapeño Peppers With Red Onion

These pickled jalapeño peppers with onions are tasty on your favorite Mexican dishes. You can also eat them by themselves, or in salads, wraps, or any dish that you want a little extra spicy kick. You can also use the pickling liquid in place of regular vinegar in homemade vinaigrettes and marinades.

Prep time: 11 minutes + 1 hour to rest
Cook time: n/a
Serves: 4

Caution: Wear gloves when handling the jalapeño peppers to prevent burning.

Ingredients
¾ cup of water
¾ cup of white vinegar
2 tablespoons kosher salt
2 tablespoons maple syrup
3-4 cloves fresh garlic, minced
1 medium red onion, sliced thin
5-6 jalapeño peppers, round slices, seeds removed

Directions
1. First, prepare the pickling liquid. Combine water, vinegar, maple syrup, minced garlic, and salt in a saucepan over medium heat. Combine the ingredients by whisking and heat until maple syrup is completely dissolved. Remove from heat and set aside.
2. Place the onion and peppers in a glass jar. Pour the pickling liquid over the contents of the jar to cover completely.

3. Let the jar sit for a minimum of one hour at room temperature and uncovered. Service immediately. You can also store in the refrigerator with a tight lid for up to one week.

Nutrition Information Per Serving*
Calories: 73
Protein: 1.6 g
Carbohydrates: 16 g
Dietary Fiber: 1.4 g
Total Sugars: 10.29 g
Fat: 0.16 g (0.03 g saturated)
* Nutritional information is provided for educational purposes only. [13]

CARAMELIZED ONIONS

While these caramelized onions require some time to prepare, you will find that they are worth it.

Prep time: 15 minutes
Cook time: approximately 1 hour
Serves: 4-6

Ingredients
3 large yellow onions
3 tablespoons coconut oil
2 tablespoons extra virgin olive oil
1/3 cup balsamic vinegar
Sea salt and black pepper

Directions

1. Remove both ends of the onion and cut it in half lengthwise. Turn one piece of onion onto the flat side and cut into thin slices, working from one end to the other. Repeat until all the onions are sliced.

2. Add the coconut oil to a large skillet over medium heat to melt. Place the onion slices in the skillet and add a small amount of olive oil. Add salt and black pepper, as desired. Stir to combine.

    Cook the onions slowly over medium heat for between 45 minutes to an hour. The actual cooking time will depend on the sugar content in the onions, the number of onions used, and their age. Stir every 5 to prevent burning.

3. Once the onions caramelized, add the balsamic vinegar to deglaze the pan. Scrape the bottom of the pan, while the liquid is bubbling, to incorporate the fond (the brown bits on the bottom of the pan) into the onions.

4. Season with extra salt and black pepper, as needed. Use immediately, or cool and store in the refrigerator for up to one week. Enjoy!

Nutrition Information Per Serving*

Calories: 141

Protein: 0.9 g

Carbohydrates: 9.4 g

Dietary Fiber: 1.6 g

Total Sugars: 5.3 g

Fat: 11.6 g (6.6 g saturated)

* Nutritional information is provided for educational purposes only. [14]

SPICY MANGO SALSA

Here's a delicious salsa with a balance of both sweet and spicy flavors.

Prep time: 10 minutes
Cook time: n/a
Serves: 4

Ingredients
2 medium mangos, peeled and chopped
1 medium red bell pepper, chopped
½ medium red onion, diced
½ medium jalapeño, minced
3 tablespoons fresh cilantro, finely chopped
2 tablespoons fresh lime juice
Sea salt and black pepper

Directions
1. Add the mango, bell pepper, red onion, jalapeño, cilantro, and lime juice in a medium bowl. Add salt and black pepper to taste. Mix the ingredients.
2. Serve or refrigerate until ready to use. Enjoy!

Nutrition Information Per Serving*
Calories: 113
Protein: 1.8 g
Carbohydrates: 28.1 g
Dietary Fiber: 3.6 g
Total Sugars: 24.6 g
Fat: 0.7 g (0.2 g saturated)

* Nutritional information is provided for educational purposes only. [14]

Healthy Vegan Cooking

CHAPTER 9 – SMOOTHIES

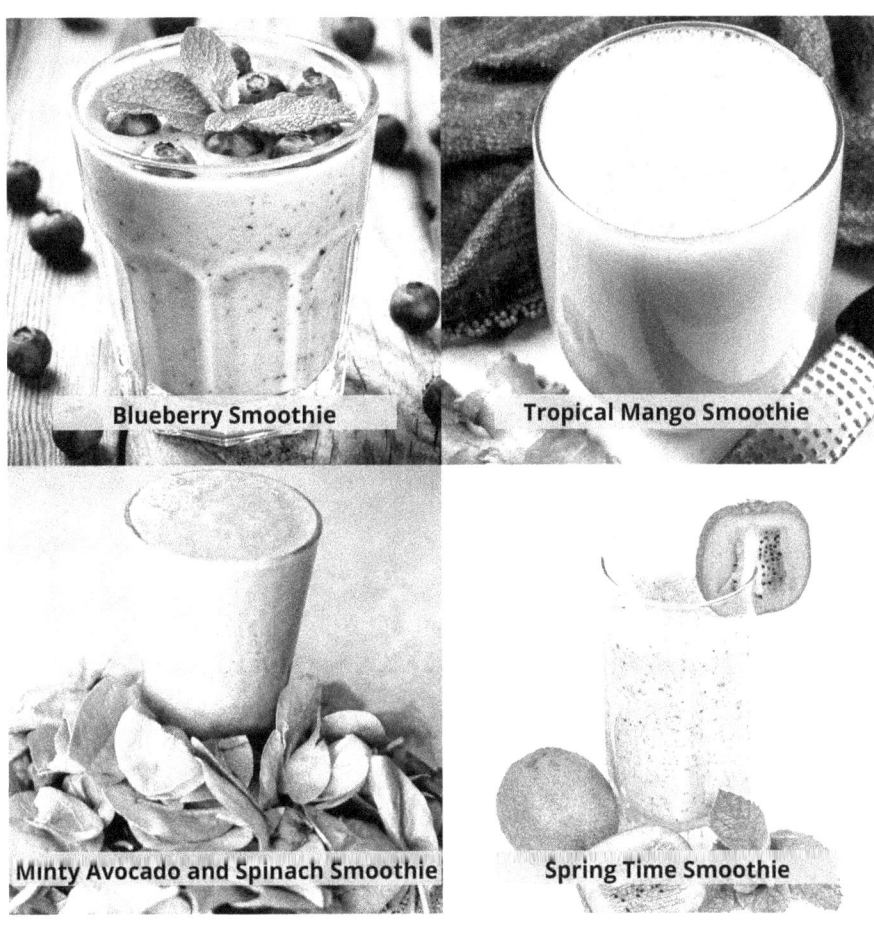

MANGO BREAKFAST SMOOTHIE

Here is a quick and easy breakfast smoothie that will make you look forward to the morning. This smoothie features the tropical flavors of coconut, mango, and pineapple. It is satisfying and refreshing.

Prep time: 10 minutes
Serves: 2

Ingredients
8 ounces coconut water
2 teaspoons fresh ginger root, finely grated
¾ cup frozen mango chunks
¾ cup frozen pineapple chunks
2 large stalks celery, cut into chunks
1/3 medium cucumber, peeled and diced into large chunks
3 tablespoons fresh lime juice
5-6 ice cubes

Directions
1. Add all the ingredients into a high-powered blender and turn on to its lowest setting. Slowly increase the speed and blend until all ingredients are smooth.
2. Pour into chilled glasses and serve. Enjoy!

Nutrition Information Per Serving*
Calories: 104
Protein: 2.1 g
Carbohydrates: 25 g
Dietary Fiber: 3.7 g
Total Sugars: 18.6 g
Fat: 0.65 g (0.3 g saturated)

* Nutritional information is provided for educational purposes only. [13]

Banana Bread and Blueberry Smoothie

Here's a quick and delicious smoothie that is great for breakfast or any time of the day.

Prep time: 7 minutes
Serves: 2

Ingredients
1 tablespoon chia seeds
3 tablespoons golden flaxseed meal
2 cup vanilla unsweetened coconut milk
¼ cup blueberries
10 drops liquid stevia
2 tablespoons MCT oil
¼ teaspoon xanthan gum
½ raw banana, medium size

Directions
1. Place the ingredients into a high-speed blender.
2. Wait a few minutes to allow the chia seeds and flax to absorb the moisture.
3. Blend for 1-2 minutes until everything is fully incorporated.
4. Serve in a couple of chilled glasses.

Nutrition Information Per Serving*
Calories: 814
Protein: 9.6 g
Carbohydrates: 29.5 g
Dietary Fiber: 12.6 g
Total Sugars: 13.71 g

Fat: 79 g (63.271 g saturated)
* Nutritional information is provided for educational purposes only. [13]

BLUEBERRY SMOOTHIE

Prep time: 5 minutes
Serves: 1

Ingredients
¼ cup blueberries
1 cup coconut milk
1 scoop plain plant-based protein powder
1 teaspoon vanilla extract
1 teaspoon MCT Oil

Directions
1. Add the ingredients into a blender.
2. Puree until it reaches the desired consistency. Add some ice if desired.

Nutrition Information Per Serving*
Calories: 395
Protein: 33 g
Carbohydrates: 30.6 g
Dietary Fiber: 3.9 g
Total Sugars: 26.5 g
Fat: 15 g (9 g saturated)
* Nutritional information is provided for educational purposes only. [13]

SPRING TIME SMOOTHIE

Here's a delicious springtime smoothie. However, it can be enjoyed at any time of the year by substituting fresh fruit for frozen fruit. Also, the plant-based protein powder gives this smoothie a nice protein boost.

Prep time: 5 minutes
Serves: 1

Ingredients
1 small wedge or 1.8 oz. honeydew or cantaloupe
¼ cup coconut milk, full-fat cream
1.8 oz. (average-sized) Avocado
1 tablespoon chia seeds
¼ cup kiwifruit/berries
¼ cup plain or vanilla plant-based protein powder (soy, oat, rice, other)
2-6 drops liquid stevia extract
½ cup water

Directions
1. Cut the avocado in half and scoop out the insides; add it to a blender.
2. Add in the kiwi, peeled melon, and the other ingredients.
3. Blend well and serve.

Nutrition Information Per Serving*
Calories: 692
Protein: 19.75 g
Carbohydrates: 42.4 g
Dietary Fiber: 21.3 g
Total Sugars: 14 g

Fat: 54.8 g (23.3 g saturated)
* Nutritional information is provided for educational purposes only. [13]

MACA ALMOND SMOOTHIE

Prep time: 5 minutes
Serves: 1

Ingredients
¾ cup unsweetened almond milk
¼ cup coconut milk
1 tablespoon unsweetened almond butter
1 tablespoon soy protein powder
1 tablespoon extra-virgin olive oil
2 teaspoons maca powder

Directions
1. Combine the ingredients in a blender.
2. Mix well until it is smooth and serve in a chilled mug or glass.

Nutrition Information Per Serving*
Calories: 446
Protein: 12.5 g
Carbohydrates: 13.8 g
Dietary Fiber: 5.7 g
Total Sugars: 4.7 g
Fat: 39.9 g (15.6 g saturated)
* Nutritional information is provided for educational purposes only. [14]

Minty Avocado and Spinach Smoothie

Prep time: 7 minutes
Serves: 1

Ingredients

1 cup fresh spinach
½ cup unsweetened almond milk
½ avocado
1 scoop plant-based protein powder (soy, oat, rice, other)
10 drops stevia
¼ teaspoon peppermint extract
1 cup ice

Directions

1. Combine the milk, spinach, avocado, stevia, protein powder, extract, and ice in a blender.
2. Mix well until creamy smooth.

Nutrition Information Per Serving*

Calories: 211
Protein: 13.1 g
Carbohydrates: 9.6 g
Dietary Fiber: 7.1 g
Total Sugars: 0.4 g
Fat: 15.2 g (2 g saturated)

* Nutritional information is provided for educational purposes only. [14]

PUMPKIN AND AVOCADO SMOOTHIE

Prep time: 5 minutes
Serves: 1

Ingredients
3 tablespoons pumpkin puree
¾ cup coconut milk, full-fat
1 tablespoon MCT oil
½ avocado
½ teaspoon pumpkin spice
1 teaspoon vanilla extract, alcohol-free

Directions
1. Add the ingredients to a blender.
2. Mix well until creamy smooth.

Nutritional Note: Pumpkin is high in beta carotene, which is converted into vitamin A in the body. This is beneficial for reducing the risk of some cancers, heart disease, and asthma. [38]

Nutrition Information Per Serving*
Calories: 688
Protein: 6.3 g
Carbohydrates: 22.3 g
Dietary Fiber: 11.5 g
Total Sugars: 8.4 g
Fat: 70.4 g (54 g saturated)

* Nutritional information is provided for educational purposes only. [14]

CHAPTER 10 – BREAKFAST

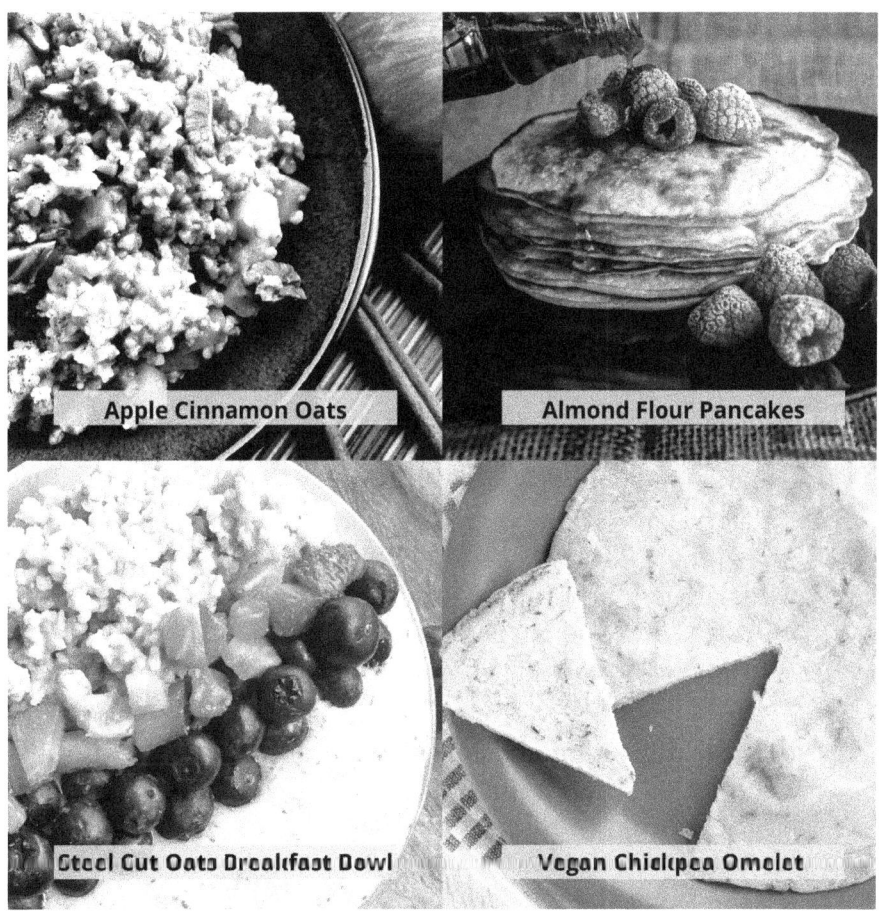

Almond Flour Pancakes

Cook Time: 20 minutes
Prep Time: 5 minutes
Servings: 2

Ingredients
1 cup almond Flour
2 tablespoons olive oil
¼ teaspoon sea salt
1 teaspoon baking powder
1 teaspoon vanilla extract
2 tablespoons soy milk
1 tablespoon monk fruit sweetener
6 tablespoons aquafaba

Directions
1. Heat a large skillet to medium-low temperature.
2. At the same time, combine the aquafaba, monk fruit sweetener, soy milk, vanilla extract, and olive oil with a whisk. Next, add in the almond flour, sea salt, and baking powder. Stir the ingredients together until there are no clumps. However, do not over-mix the batter. Otherwise, they won't be fluffy.
3. Grease the preheated skillet with either vegan butter or coconut oil, then pour the pancake batter into little disks, each pancake containing 3 to 4 tablespoons each. Or measure out the batter using a ¼ cup to ensure they are all the same size.
4. Allow the pancakes to cook until they begin to set up and bubbles begin to form. Once they are sturdy, use a spatula and gently flip them over. Each side should only need to cook for about three to four minutes. However,

watch the pancakes closely because they can burn quickly if your stove is too hot.

5. Once the pancakes are done, remove them from the skillet. Repeat until all the pancakes are done. It should yield about six smalls to medium pancakes, perfect for two individuals. Enjoy the pancakes with fruit, sweetened coconut cream, or maple syrup.

Nutrition Information Per Serving*

Calories: 162
Protein: 0.61 g
Carbohydrates: 7.55 g
Dietary Fiber: 0.1 g
Total Sugars: 5.7 g
Fat: 14.3 g (2.2 g saturated)

* Nutritional information is provided for educational purposes only. [13]

SLOW COOKER APPLE-CINNAMON OATS

This recipe cooks overnight, so you won't need to rush to prepare breakfast in the morning. And, you will wake to your house smelling like a delicious baked apple pie.

Prep time: 15 minutes
Cook time: 6-8 hours
Serves: 4-6

Important Tips

1. Do not substitute any other type of oats for this recipe. The cooking times are for steel-cut oats only.
2. It very important to either line or heavily grease the sides of the slow cooker crock before preparing this recipe. If

you skip this step, the oats will stick to the sides and it will be very difficult to clean.

Ingredients

1 cup steel-cut oats

3 cups water

1 cup fresh apple cider

2 medium apples, cored and diced

1½ tablespoons maple syrup

1 teaspoon ground cinnamon

½ teaspoon ground nutmeg

½ teaspoon ground allspice

½ teaspoon salt

To serve

1 medium apple, cored and diced

½ cup pecans, chopped

maple syrup

Directions

1. Grease or line a slow cooker crock. Add the oats, apples, cider, water, maple syrup, nutmeg, cinnamon, allspice, and salt. Stir to combine.

2. Cook on low for about 6 to 8 hours. Actual cooking time will vary depending on the slow cooker you're using, so check for doneness after 5 hours and adjust cooking time accordingly.

3. Once done, allow it to cool slightly before spooning into bowls. You can top them with fresh chopped apples, pecans, and some maple syrup if desired.

Nutrition Information Per Serving*
Calories: 300
Protein: 6.6 g
Carbohydrates: 51.3 g
Dietary Fiber: 7.4 g
Total Sugars: 24 g
Fat: 9.6 g (1.1 g saturated)
* Nutritional information is provided for educational purposes only. [13]

INSTANT POT STEEL-CUT OATS WITH BERRIES

This is a healthy breakfast that is easy to make. The great thing about the Instant Pot is that you can get it started and forget about it while it cooks.

Time Saving Tip
Prepare the yogurt mixture ahead of time so that everything is ready for breakfast. Also, use frozen blueberries and strawberries to reduce the preparation time.

Prep time: 10 minutes
Cook time: 25 minutes + time to come to pressure
Serves: 4

Ingredients
Non-stick cooking spray
1 cup steel-cut oats
3¼ cups water
2 cups coconut yogurt
1½ tablespoons chia seeds
1 tablespoon real maple syrup, and extra for serving

1 cup strawberries, hulled and quartered

1 cup fresh blueberries, rinsed and dried

Directions
1. Apply a non-stick cooking spray to the Instant Pot cooking container.
2. Add the steel-cut oats and water and stir to mix.
3. Now prepare the Instant Pot for cooking. Cover it and lock the lid into position. Move the pressure valve to the "Sealing" position. Press the "Manual" button and set it on high heat. Set the cooking time to 10 minutes.
4. Prepare the yogurt mixture while oats are cooking. Add the yogurt, maple syrup, and chia seeds in a small bowl and stir to mix. Set aside.
5. When the cooking is done, turn off the Instant Pot immediately to prevent burning. Allow the pressure to release for about 15 minutes. Then perform a quick release for any remaining pressure.
6. Carefully remove the lid. Stir the oats to combine. Transfer the oats to the serving bowls. Add a little more oats on one half of the bowl and add the yogurt mixture on the other side.
7. Place the strawberries and blueberries between the two sides. Serve immediately. You can add extra maple syrup on the side if desired.

Nutrition Information Per Serving*
Calories: 152

Protein: 6.3 g

Carbohydrates: 33.6 g

Dietary Fiber: 8.3 g

Total Sugars: 11.9 g

Fat: 3.8 g (0.7 g saturated)

* Nutritional information is provided for educational purposes only. [13]

VEGAN CHICKPEA OMELET

Prep time: 5 minutes
Cook time: 5 minutes
Serves: 2

Ingredients
3 heaping tablespoons chickpea flour
½ teaspoon salt
pinch ground black pepper
8 tablespoons water
1 small onion, chopped
2 tablespoons avocado oil
Bunch of fresh herbs (dill, basil, others as desired), chopped

Directions
1. Place chickpea flour, salt, and pepper in a mixing bowl and whisk. Next, add the water to the mixture and whisk until creamy.
2. Add the chopped onion and chopped herbs and mix.
3. Add the avocado oil to a pan and heat.
4. Spoon the batter into the hot pan in a round shape.
5. Cook uncovered for a few minutes.
6. Flip omelet over with a spatula and cook for a few more minutes.
7. Remove from heat, cut it, and serve. It can be served with or without bread. Add vegetables and fruit for a healthy and balanced breakfast.

Nutrition Information Per Serving*
Calories: 196
Protein: 4.3 g

Carbohydrates: 13.3 g
Dietary Fiber: 2.9 g
Total Sugars: 2.6 g
Fat: 15.1 g (1.7 g saturated)

* Nutritional information is provided for educational purposes only. [14]

CHAPTER 11 – SOUPS AND STOCK

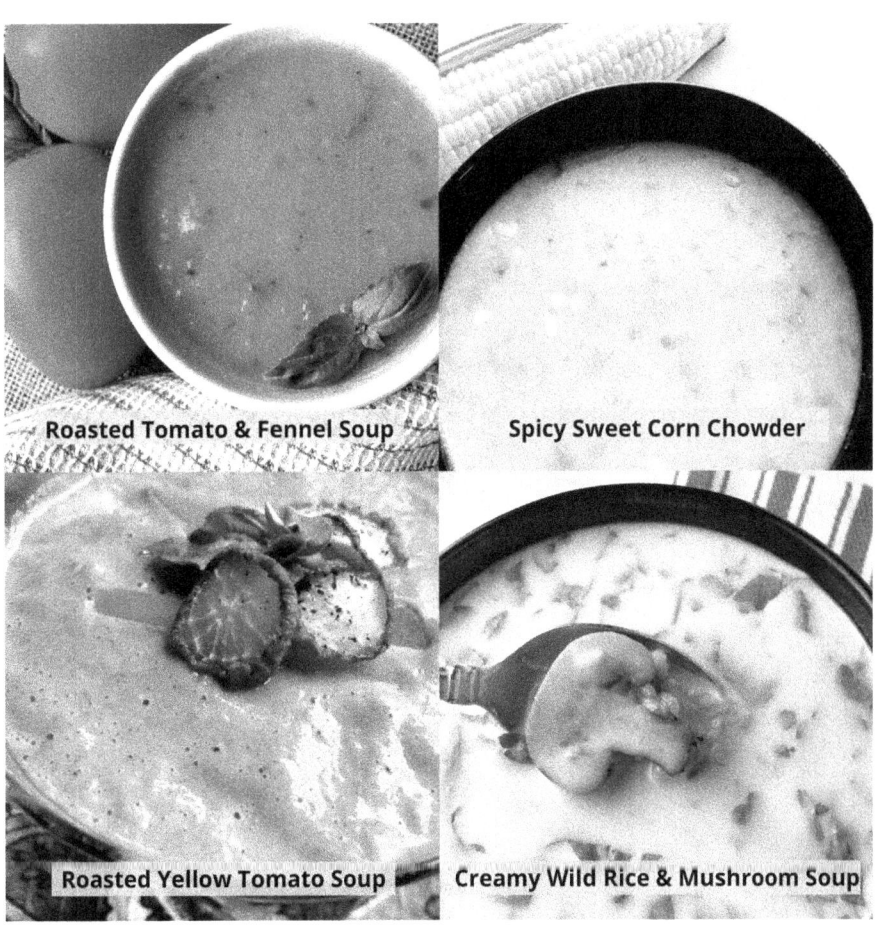

CREAMY WILD RICE AND MUSHROOM SOUP

This soup is satisfying and comforting. The pureed cannellini beans and the coconut milk give this soup a delicious and creamy texture. The minced and chopped vegetables provide a flavor that is consistent throughout.

Prep time: 20 minutes
Cook time: 3-8 hours
Serves: 4-6

Ingredients
1 cup multi-color wild rice blend, uncooked
1 small white onion, roughly chopped
3 stalks celery, roughly chopped
2 large carrots, peeled and chopped
3-4 cloves garlic, peeled
12 ounces fresh mushrooms, washed, divided
one 15-ounce can cannellini beans, undrained
1 whole bay leaf
2 teaspoons garlic powder
6-8 cups vegetable stock, divided
½ cup full-fat coconut milk
¼ cup fresh parsley, finely chopped
Salt and black pepper

Tip
Rinse and drain the beans before pureeing them to reduce the amount of salt.

Directions

1. Rinse the rice with running cold water until the water is clear. Let the rice drain. Then, place the rice into a 5 or 6 slow cooker.
2. Add the celery, onion, carrots, and garlic to a food processor. Pulse until the content is very finely minced and transfer to slow cooker crock.
3. Add 2/3 of the mushrooms to the food processor and pulse until finely chopped. Finely slice the remaining mushrooms. Add both chopped and sliced mushrooms to the slow cooker.
4. Add the cannellini beans and a little water to the food processor and puree until smooth. Pour into slow cooker crock with other ingredients, then add bay leaf, garlic powder, and 6 cups of vegetable stock. Add salt and black pepper as desired. Stir and thoroughly combine the ingredients.
5. Put the cover on the slow cooker. Cook on the high setting for about 3-4 hours or cook on the low setting for 6-8 hours. The actual cooking time may vary by individual slow cookers. So check for doneness after 2½ hours (or 5½ hours for low) and adjust cooking time as needed. When the rice is done, it should be tender and not mushy.
6. Once the soup is done cooking, remove and discard the bay leaf. Add the chopped parsley, coconut milk, and the extra vegetable stock, if needed, to achieve the desired consistency.
7. Season with more salt and black pepper, to taste, and stir to combine thoroughly. Serve immediately and enjoy!

Nutrition Information Per Serving*

Calories: 161
Protein: 7.4 g

Carbohydrates: 26 g
Dietary Fiber: 6.6 g
Total Sugars: 6.3 g
Fat: 2.1 g (1.1 g saturated)
* Nutritional information is provided for educational purposes only. [14]

Chilled Cucumber Avocado Soup with Fresh Dill

This easy and refreshing chilled soup is ideal for a hot summer day. It only requires a few minutes of preparation time, and you don't even need to turn on your oven or cooktop.

Prep time: 15 minutes + 2-3 hrs refrigeration time
Cook time: n/a
Serves: 4

Ingredients
½ cup vegetable stock
2 large cucumbers, peeled and cubed
1½ cups coconut yogurt
½ medium avocado, peeled and seeded
1 medium shallot, peeled and halved
3 tablespoons fresh dill, chopped
2 tablespoons fresh lime juice
2 teaspoons ground cumin
2 teaspoons sea salt
Black pepper
optional: sprigs of fresh dill or sliced cucumber for garnish

Directions

1. Add the ingredients to a blender or food processor and blend until smooth. For a thinner soup, add a little more vegetable stock until you reach the desired consistency. Adjust seasonings to taste.
2. Cover and refrigerate for at least 2-3 hours before serving.
3. Serve chilled topped with sprigs of fresh dill and thin slices of cucumber. Enjoy!

Nutrition Information Per Serving*

Calories: 175
Protein: 6.8 g
Carbohydrates: 22 g
Dietary Fiber: 3 g
Total Sugars: 14.8 g
Fat: 6.6 g (3.3 g saturated)

* Nutritional information is provided for educational purposes only. [14]

CREAMY BROCCOLI SOUP

Prep Time: 3 minutes
Cook Time: 30 minutes
Servings: 6

Ingredients

6 cups broccoli, chopped
5 cloves garlic, minced
2 ribs celery, chopped
1½ teaspoons sea salt

1 cup soy milk

1 teaspoon onion powder

3 cups vegetable broth

2 tablespoons olive oil

½ teaspoon black pepper, ground

Directions

1. Add olive oil and celery to a pot on medium heat and allow it to cook for a few minutes until the celery becomes tender. Next, add the minced garlic and seasonings, and allow them to cook for 1-2 more minutes or until the garlic becomes fragrant. Watch carefully so you don't burn the garlic.
2. Add the soy milk and broth to the pot. Allow the ingredients to simmer for about 20 minutes until the broccoli is tender.
3. Allow the broccoli soup to cool for a few minutes and then place it into a blender and pulse it until it is smooth. **Caution** is warranted if the soup is still hot. The pressure from the steam can build up and cause the blender lid to pop off if there is no ventilation. You can either blend the soup until completely smooth or leave it slightly chunky.
4. Serve the soup immediately or reheat it on the stove before serving.

Nutrition Information Per Serving*

Calories: 118

Protein: 6.5 g

Carbohydrates: 10.4 g

Dietary Fiber: 2.8 g

Total Sugars: 3.7 g

Fat: 6.4 g (0.9 g saturated)

* Nutritional information is provided for educational purposes only. [14]

GARLIC CASTILIAN SOUP

Prep Time: 10 minutes
Cook Time: 35 minutes
Servings: 4

Ingredients
3 large cloves garlic
2 tablespoons olive oil
3 cups vegetable broth
3 cups water
1 thinly sliced red bell pepper
Salt and pepper

Directions
1. Add the olive oil to a large saucepan and heat on medium. Add the garlic cloves to the pan and sauté for 3 minutes.
2. Add 1 cup of vegetable broth. Cover and simmer for 10 minutes.
3. Use a fork to mash the garlic into a paste.
4. Add the water and the remaining vegetable broth. Bring to a boil and then add the red bell pepper. Simmer 15 minutes.
5. Cook approximately 4 minutes until solid. Serve immediately.

Nutrition Information Per Serving*
Calories: 84
Protein: 0.4 g
Carbohydrates: 5.2 g
Dietary Fiber: 1.2 g

Total Sugars: 3 g
Fat: 7.1 g (1 g saturated)
* Nutritional information is provided for educational purposes only. [14]

ROASTED YELLOW TOMATO SOUP

Summer and fall are the ideal times to enjoy this easy to make roasted yellow tomato soup. Use tomatoes of the same color for a better presentation. Mixing yellow and red tomatoes will result in an unattractive hue that isn't very appetizing. Also, slow roasting the tomatoes will bring out their natural sweetness. However, this will cause browning that will result in a darker soup than if you use raw tomatoes.

Prep time: 15-20 min
Cook time: 2 ½ – 3 hours
Serves: 4-6

Soup Ingredients
Ripe yellow tomatoes, approximately 2 pounds
1 tablespoon garlic powder
½ cup vegetable stock
1 large bunch of fresh basil, washed and patted dry
1 medium yellow onion, peeled and quartered
2 celery stalks, washed and cut into big pieces
2 large or 3 small cloves of garlic, peeled
1 tablespoon ground cumin
3 tablespoons full fat coconut milk
Freshly cracked black pepper and sea salt

Garnish Ingredients
1 large bunch red radishes
several very thin slices of yellow tomato
sprigs fresh basil

Directions
1. Preheat oven to 300 °F.
2. Place parchment paper on a large rimmed baking sheet and set aside.
3. Slice yellow tomatoes into ½" slices and place on the prepared baking sheet, leaving a small space between the slices. Sprinkle tomatoes with salt, pepper and garlic powder.
4. Place the baking sheet with the tomatoes in the preheated oven and roast the tomatoes for about 2 hours or until the tomatoes are brown around the edges.
5. Wash and pat the radishes dry before cutting into thin slices*. Place the radish slices on a lined baking sheet and sprinkle with salt and black pepper, as desired. Place in the oven with the tomatoes. Check them frequently because they will brown up much faster than the tomatoes. Roast the radishes until they are slightly browned and crispy. Remove them from the oven and use them to garnish the finished soup.

    *For best results, use a mandoline slicer for radishes to achieve even thickness.

6. Once the tomatoes are done roasting, remove them from the oven and let them cool slightly. Next, add the roasted tomato slices, stock, onion, basil, celery, garlic, cumin, and coconut milk to a high-powered blender or a food processor. Season with salt and cracked black pepper as desired.
7. Blend on high until thoroughly combined and smooth. Taste and add more seasonings if needed. If desired, add

more vegetable stock, 1 tablespoon at a time, and re-blend to achieve the desired consistency.
8. Serve the soup topped with roasted radishes and a sprig of fresh basil. Enjoy!

Nutrition Information Per Serving*
Calories: 102
Protein: 2.9 g
Carbohydrates: 16.1 g
Dietary Fiber: 2.8 g
Total Sugars: 8.5 g
Fat: 3.8 g (2.6 g saturated)
* Nutritional information is provided for educational purposes only. [14]

ROASTED TOMATOES AND FENNEL SOUP

This healthy, dairy-free roasted vegetable soup is great for cold or chilly days. It also tastes great the next day, so you may want to make a double or triple batch. This soup can be stored in the refrigerator for two to three days. It can also be frozen for a quick meal or a tasty snack on those hectic days.

Prep time: 10 minutes
Cook time: 35 minutes
Serves: 4

Tip
A blender can be used in place of a stick or immersion blender for blending the cooked vegetables and liquid. However, to prevent the hot liquid from building up pressure and exploding, ensure that the blender lid is properly vented.

Healthy Vegan Cooking

Ingredients

1½ pounds Roma tomatoes, halved
2 medium red bell peppers, remove the seeds and quarter
1 large fennel bulb, thinly sliced
2 large carrots, cut in half lengthwise
2 medium shallots, skin removed and halved
4 cloves garlic, smashed and peeled
2 tablespoons extra virgin olive oil
2 tablespoons fresh thyme leaves
4 cups organic vegetable broth
½ cup full-fat coconut milk
½ cup fresh basil leaves, thinly sliced
Sea salt and black pepper

Directions

1. Preheat the oven to 400 °F and place parchment paper on a large, rimmed baking sheet. Set aside.
2. Place the tomatoes, fennel, carrots, red peppers, garlic, and shallots in a single layer on the baking sheet. Next, drizzle with the olive oil. Then, season with salt and pepper to your taste. Mix the veggies and sprinkle them with the thyme leaves.
3. Place the baking sheet into the oven. Roast until the vegetables are tender and lightly charred, about 20-25 minutes.
4. Transfer the roasted veggies and juices from the baking sheet to a large soup pot and add the vegetable broth. Cook over medium heat until the soup is bubbling hot. Stir occasionally. Remove from heat.
5. Using a blender, blend the ingredients in the pot until it is completely smooth. Stir in the basil and coconut milk and serve.

Nutrition Information Per Serving*
Calories: 231
Protein: 3 g
Carbohydrates: 25.8 g
Dietary Fiber: 5.1 g
Total Sugars: 11.6 g
Fat: 13.4 g (6.5 g saturated)
* Nutritional information is provided for educational purposes only. [14]

Spicy Sweet Corn Chowder

Prep time: 20 minutes
Cook time: 30-40 minutes
Serves: 6

Tip
Extreme caution is warranted when blending hot liquids since they could explode. Cool the liquid some and ensure that the lid on the blender is properly ventilated before blending.

Ingredients
2 tablespoons extra virgin olive oil
2 stalks celery, finely chopped
2 large carrots, finely chopped
1 medium white onion, finely chopped
4 cloves fresh garlic, finely minced
1 jalapeño pepper, finely chopped
5 cups organic vegetable stock
2½ pounds Russet potatoes, chopped
5 ears sweet corn, kernels only
1 tablespoon fresh oregano

2 teaspoons ground cumin

1 bay leaf

½ cup almond or full-fat coconut milk

Sea salt and black pepper

Optional: fresh chives to garnish

Directions
1. Wash and pat dry the vegetables before prepping. You can either peel the potatoes or leave the skin on, as desired.
2. Heat the olive oil in a large, deep skillet over medium heat, then add the carrots, celery, onion, garlic, and jalapeño pepper to the skillet. Sauté the ingredients for a few minutes. Stir consistently, until vegetables are soft and fragrant.
3. Pour the vegetable stock into skillet. Then, add the sweet corn, potatoes, cumin, oregano, and bay leaf. Season with salt and pepper, as needed, and stir to combine.
4. Reduce the heat to medium-low and simmer. Cook uncovered until heated throughout, and the potatoes are tender approximately 20 minutes. Stir occasionally while cooking.
5. Transfer 3-4 cups of the soup mixture to a blender or food processor and blend until smooth. (See tip above first!). Pour the pureed soup mixture back into the skillet and stir to combine. Taste and adjust seasonings, as desired.
6. Add the almond or coconut milk to the skillet. Stir and simmer for about 5-10 more minutes to heat thoroughly. Remove the bay leaf before serving. Enjoy!

Nutrition Information Per Serving*

Calories: 701

Protein: 16.6 g

Carbohydrates: 147.5 g
Dietary Fiber: 22.7 g
Total Sugars: 16.3 g
Fat: 7.6 g (2 g saturated)
* Nutritional information is provided for educational purposes only. [14]

HOMEMADE VEGETABLE STOCK

This vegetable stock is so quick and easy to make. It is a great way to use up extra vegetables and herbs before they spoil. Extra stock can be frozen for quick and easy soups and stews. It can also be used in your slow cooker meals.

Prep time: 25 minutes
Yield: 4 cups

Ingredients
¼ cup olive oil
2 large onions, peeled and cut into large chunks
4 cloves garlic, peeled and smashed
3 large carrots, cut into chunks
3 stalks celery, cut into chunks
water to cover
8 sprigs fresh thyme
4 sprigs fresh rosemary
1 bay leaf
1 handful whole fresh parsley
small handful whole peppercorns

Directions

1. Add olive oil to a large stockpot and heat over medium-high heat. Add garlic, onions, celery, and carrots to the heated oil. Sauté for about 5-6 minutes.
2. Add enough water to cover the vegetables. Then add the thyme, rosemary, bay leaf, parsley, and peppercorns. Heat the mixture over medium-high heat until it just about boils. Then reduce the heat to medium-low. Stir it and allow it to simmer, uncovered, for approximately an hour.
3. Place a stainless steel colander over a large pot in the sink. Pour the contents of the stockpot into the colander to separate the solids from the liquid. Discard the solids. Allow the stock to cool completely and then transfer it to storage containers for freezing. Freeze until ready to use.

CHAPTER 12 – SALADS

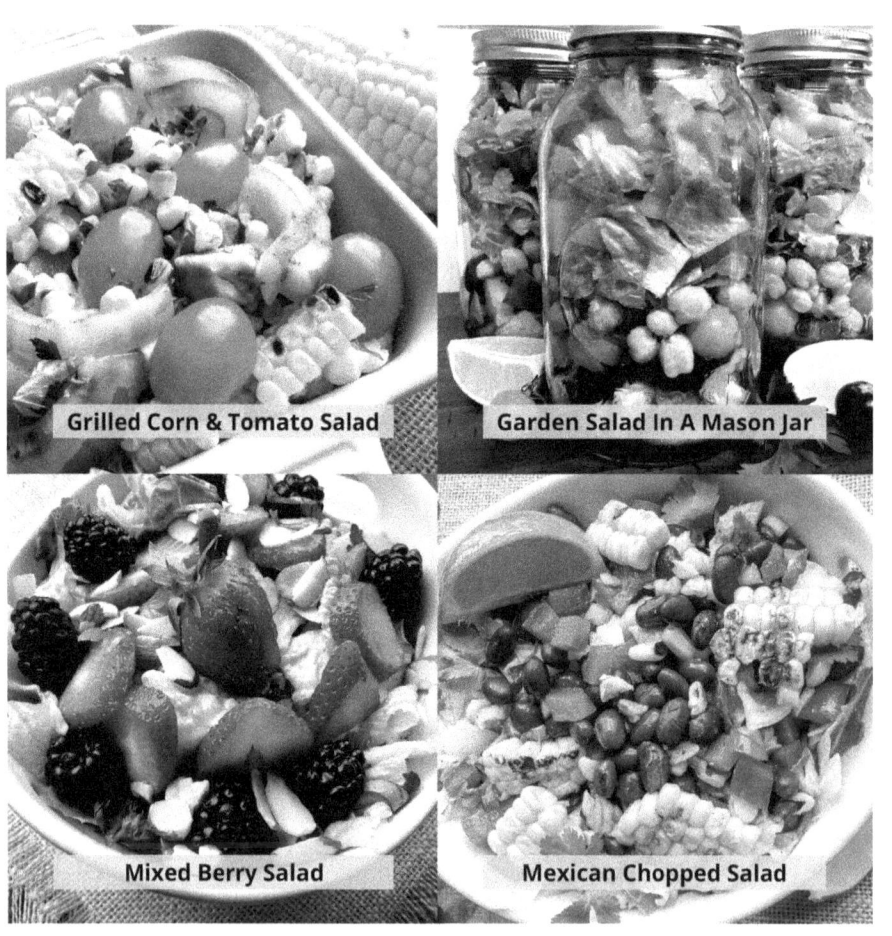

Mixed Berry Salad with Raspberry Vinaigrette

The combination of fresh berries and mint give this salad a great, fresh taste.

Prep time: 15 minutes
Cook time: none
Serves: 4

Ingredients
1/4 cup rice wine vinegar
1/3 cup fresh raspberries, washed
2 teaspoons fresh lemon juice
1/2 cup extra virgin olive oil
1/2 teaspoon sea salt
1 head Romaine lettuce, washed and remove stem, chopped
1/3 cup fresh mint, chopped
1 cup fresh strawberries, washed and hulled, sliced
1 cup fresh blackberries, washed
1/3 cup sliced almonds, toasted

Directions
1. Chill salad plates in the refrigerator while preparing this recipe.
2. Add vinegar, raspberries, lemon juice, and olive oil to a food processor and blend until smooth. Add salt. Set aside.
3. Add the lettuce, mint, strawberries, blackberries, and toasted almonds into a bowl and toss gently until combined.
4. Add raspberry vinaigrette as desired and serve immediately on the chilled salad plates.

Nutrition Information Per Serving*
Calories: 303
Protein: 2.9 g
Carbohydrates: 13 g
Dietary Fiber: 6.8 g
Total Sugars: 5.96 g
Fat: 27.9 g (3.8 g saturated)
* Nutritional information is provided for educational purposes only. [13]

GARDEN SALAD IN A MASON JAR WITH BALSAMIC DRESSING

Salads in mason jars are great for on the go lunches and easy for dinners. It is best to add the dressing first, followed by the harder vegetables that won't become soggy from the dressing. Then add the softer vegetables and legumes. Finally, add the leafy green vegetables and herbs on top. You can also add other ingredients such as rice, pasta, beans, or nuts, or other toppings as desired.

Prep time: 30 minutes
Cook time: n/a
Serves: 6

Special Equipment
6 quart-sized mason jars

Basic Balsamic Dressing
2/3 cup extra virgin olive oil
1/3 cup balsamic vinegar
2 tablespoons Dijon mustard

2 teaspoons fresh oregano leaves
3 tablespoons fresh lime juice
1 tablespoon maple syrup
Sea salt and black pepper

Salad Ingredients
2 medium English cucumbers, chopped
2 large bell peppers, seeded, chopped
one 15-oz. can chickpeas, rinsed, drained
1 cup grape or cherry tomatoes, halved
2 heads Romaine lettuce, chopped
½ cup fresh parsley leaves, chopped
½ cup fresh basil leaves, chopped

Directions
1. First, prepare the dressing. Whisk the olive oil, vinegar, mustard, lime juice, and maple syrup together in a small glass or stainless steel bowl. Add salt and pepper as desired. Set aside.
2. Wash and pat dry the vegetables before prepping. In a medium bowl, combine the romaine lettuce, parsley, and basil. Divide all vegetables into 6 equal portions. Set aside.
3. Divide the dressing among the six mason jars. Start by adding a layer of cucumbers to each jar. Then add a layer of bell peppers. Next, add the chickpeas and then the tomatoes. Finally, add the lettuce and herb mixture on top. Seal each jar with a lid.
4. Store the salad jars in the refrigerator until ready to serve. Each salad will last 4-5 days. The salad may be eaten from the jar on the go, or it can be served in a salad bowl.

Nutrition Information Per Serving*
Calories: 399
Protein: 9.1 g
Carbohydrates: 34 g
Dietary Fiber: 10.5 g
Total Sugars: 12.56 g
Fat: 27 g (3.6 g saturated)
* Nutritional information is provided for educational purposes only. [13]

ROASTED BEETS, CITRUS, AND FENNEL SALAD

This salad has tender roasted beets and a blend of citrus and fennel for a light and satisfying meal. It is also great when paired with a delicious bowl of hot or cold soup.

Prep time: 10 minutes
Cook time: 45 minutes – 1 hour
Serves: 6

Orange Vinaigrette Ingredients
¼ cup balsamic vinegar
1 teaspoon fresh orange zest
2 tablespoons fresh orange juice
1 teaspoon fresh lemon zest
1 tablespoon fresh lemon juice
1 tablespoon fresh lime juice
¼ cup rice wine vinegar
½ cup extra virgin olive oil
1 tablespoon maple syrup
2 teaspoons Dijon mustard

1 clove garlic, finely minced
Sea salt and black pepper

Salad Ingredients
4 medium beets
3 tablespoons extra virgin olive oil
2 large oranges, zested, sliced, and cut into wedges
½ small fennel bulb, thinly sliced
2 cups baby arugula lettuce
2 cups mixed salad greens
½ cup walnuts, chopped

Directions
1. Preheat oven to 400 °F.
2. Combine the vinaigrette ingredients in a glass bowl and whisk together thoroughly to combine. Set aside.
3. Wash the beets and pat dry. Place each beet onto a separate piece of aluminum foil, then rub it with olive oil. Generously salt each beet before wrapping in aluminum foil and placing it on a rimmed baking sheet.
4. Place the baking sheet into the preheated oven and roast the beets for 45 minutes to an hour or until the beets are tender.
5. Remove from oven and set aside to cool slightly. When the beets are cool enough to handle, peel them under cool running water and then cut them into slices.
6. Toss the arugula and mixed greens together with a little vinaigrette in a large bowl. Place the greens onto either a serving platter or chilled individual salad plates. Top the greens with roasted beets, orange slices, fennel slices, and chopped walnuts.
7. Garnish with wispy fennel fronds, if desired, and serve immediately with the remaining salad dressing. Enjoy!

Nutrition Information Per Serving*
Calories: 353
Protein: 3.6 g
Carbohydrates: 21 g
Dietary Fiber: 7 g
Total Sugars: 14.94 g
Fat: 29.5 g (3.8 g saturated)
* Nutritional information is provided for educational purposes only. [13]

Mexican Chopped Salad with Avocado Dressing

This fresh Mexican chopped salad is filling enough to serve as a light main course on its own. You can also serve this salad with soup for a complete meal. This healthy and delicious salad has lots of veggies, black beans, and herbs.

Prep time: 10 minutes
Cook time: 8 minutes
Serves: 4

Tip
One cup of cooked frozen sweet corn can be used when fresh corn is not available. In this case, just skip directions 2-3 below.

Creamy Avocado Dressing Ingredients
1 large avocado, pitted
½ small shallot, peeled and halved
3 tablespoons fresh cilantro, chopped
¼ cup plain coconut yogurt
2 tablespoons extra virgin olive oil
2 tablespoons fresh lime juice

2 teaspoons real maple syrup
Optional: 2-3 tablespoons water, if needed
Sea salt and black pepper

Chopped Salad Ingredients
2 large ears of corn, husks and silk removed
1 tablespoon extra virgin olive oil
1 head iceberg lettuce, chopped
2 cups fresh arugula, chopped
¼ cup fresh cilantro, finely chopped
1 medium red bell pepper, diced
½ medium red onion, diced
one 15-oz. can black beans, rinsed and drained
2 tablespoons fresh lime juice
1 teaspoon ground cumin
1 large lime, cut into 8 wedges
Sea salt and black pepper

Directions
1. Prepare the dressing by combining all the ingredients in a blender or food processor and blending until smooth. Add a small amount of water, as needed, to yield the desired consistency. Taste and adjust seasonings as desired. Place the dressing in the refrigerator until the salad is ready to serve.
2. Brush the corn with olive oil. For outdoor cooking, place it on a preheated gas grill over medium direct heat. For cooking indoors, place it on a grill pan, sprayed with non-stick cooking spray, over medium-high heat.
3. Cook the corn until the kernels are slightly charred. Rotate one-quarter turn every couple of minutes until each side is done. Remove corn from the heat and cut

kernels off the cob with a knife. Save the kernels and discard the cobs. Set aside.

4. Add the arugula, iceberg lettuce, and the cilantro to a large salad bowl and toss lightly to mix. Set aside.
5. In a large mixing bowl, combine the diced bell pepper, red onion, black beans, roasted corn kernels, lime juice, and ground cumin. Add salt and black pepper, as desired. Toss lightly to combine.
6. Add the black bean mixture to the bowl with the chopped lettuce and toss gently to combine. Serve with the avocado dressing or your favorite salad dressing. Enjoy!

Nutrition Information Per Serving*
Calories: 381
Protein: 13.6 g
Carbohydrates: 39 g
Dietary Fiber: 17.9 g
Total Sugars: 9.1 g
Fat: 22.3 g (4.1 g saturated)
* Nutritional information is provided for educational purposes only. [14]

GRILLED CORN AND CHERRY TOMATO SALAD

This healthy and colorful side dish pairs well with just about any main course. It can also be served with a hearty soup for lunch.

Prep time: 10 minutes
Cook time: 10 minutes
Serves: 4

Tip
If fresh corn is not available, substitute 1 cup of frozen sweet corn. Prepare the corn according to the package instructions.

Ingredients
2 large ears fresh corn, husks and silk removed
1 tablespoon extra virgin olive oil
1 medium red onion, cut in half and in thick slices
1 pound cherry or grape tomatoes, halved
1 large avocado, chopped
¼ cup fresh parsley, roughly chopped
3 tablespoons fresh lime juice
Sea salt and black pepper

Directions
1. Brush the olive oil onto the corn. For outdoor cooking, place the corn and red onion slices on a preheated gas grill over medium direct heat. For indoor cooking, place the corn and red onion slices on a preheated grill pan sprayed with non-stick cooking spray over medium-high heat.
2. Cook corn until kernels are slightly charred. Rotate one-quarter turn every couple of minutes until each side is done. Turn red onion over once while the corn is cooking. Next, remove the vegetables from the heat and slice the kernels from the cob with a sharp knife. Transfer the onions and corn kernels to a large salad bowl. Set aside.
3. Add the avocado, tomatoes, parsley, and lime juice to the bowl. Add salt and black pepper, to taste, and toss gently to combine. Serve immediately with your main dish. Enjoy!

Nutrition Information Per Serving*

Calories: 237

Protein: 4.3 g

Carbohydrates: 29.8 g

Dietary Fiber: 5.8 g

Total Sugars: 8 g

Fat: 13.5 g (2.6 g saturated)

* Nutritional information is provided for educational purposes only. [14]

CHAPTER 13 – SIDE DISHES AND SNACKS

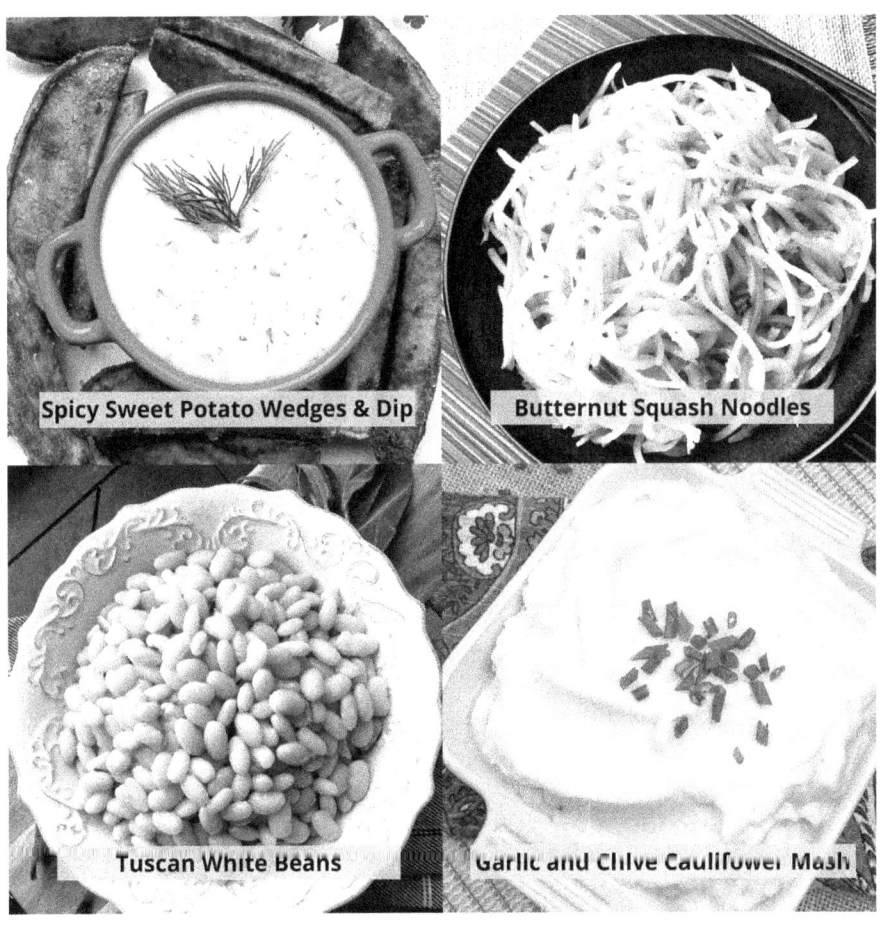

Mashed Cauliflower With Garlic and Chives

This flavorful cauliflower mash only takes about 30 minutes to make. It is a perfect side dish for those busy weeknights when you want to get a healthy dinner on the table without too much effort.

Prep time: 10 minutes
Cook time: 15-20 minutes
Serves: 4

Tip
If you steam the garlic with the cauliflower it will reduce its strong flavor.

Ingredients
1 medium cauliflower head, florets only
2-3 whole garlic cloves, peeled
2 tablespoons extra virgin olive oil
2 tablespoons unsweetened almond milk
1 teaspoon garlic powder
1 teaspoon onion powder
3 tablespoons fresh chives, chopped
Sea salt and black pepper

Directions
1. Put the cauliflower florets and garlic into a steamer basket over a pot of gently boiling water. Cover and steam until the cauliflower florets are tender, about 15-20 minutes.
2. Move the steamed cauliflower and garlic to a food processor or blender. Then add almond milk, olive oil, garlic powder, and onion powder. Add salt and black

pepper, as desired. Blend until the contents are smooth and creamy. Taste and season, as needed.
3. Transfer to a serving bowl and top with fresh chives before serving. Enjoy!

Nutrition Information Per Serving*

Calories: 74
Protein: 1.1 g
Carbohydrates: 2.8 g
Dietary Fiber: 1 g
Total Sugars: 1.3 g
Fat: 7.1 g (1 g saturated)

* Nutritional information is provided for educational purposes only. [14]

CURRIED CAULIFLOWER MASH

Prep Time: 5 min
Cook Time: 10 min
Serves: 2

Ingredients

1 medium cauliflower head, chopped

2/3 cups vegetable broth

2 garlic cloves, pressed

2 tablespoons coconut milk

1 teaspoon salt

¾ teaspoon curry powder

1 teaspoon vegan butter

Directions

1. Add cauliflower, salt, garlic, and broth to a pan.

2. Simmer covered until cauliflower is fully tender, approximately 10 minutes.
3. Add coconut milk, vegan butter, and curry.
4. Puree with an immersion blender.
5. Transfer to a serving bowl and serve. Enjoy!

Nutrition Information Per Serving*

Calories: 143
Protein: 7.9 g
Carbohydrates: 17.8 g
Dietary Fiber: 7.8 g
Total Sugars: 7.7 g
Fat: 6.3 g (4 g saturated)

* Nutritional information is provided for educational purposes only. [14]

SAVORY BUTTERNUT SQUASH NOODLES

Prepackaged convenience foods, like noodles made from heavily processed flours, are not the best options for maintaining a healthy diet.

However, this recipe features a time-savings ingredient that won't have a negative impact on your health. You can find prepackaged butternut squash "noodles" in most larger grocery stores. They are great for those nights when you are pressed for time and need to get dinner on the table quickly.

You can also make the butternut squash noodles yourself if you have a vegetable spiralizer. It only takes a few minutes. In either case, you will love this quick and delicious dish!

Prep time: 5 minutes
Cooking time: 8 minutes
Serves: 4-6

Ingredients

¼ cup extra virgin olive oil, divided

4 cups prepackaged butternut squash noodles

2 tablespoons fresh sage, chopped

2 teaspoons ground cinnamon

Sea salt and black pepper

Directions

1. Add two tablespoons of olive oil to a large skillet over medium heat. Add the noodles and cook for about 4 to 5 minutes. Turn them frequently, so they cook evenly. Once the noodles are tender, remove them from the pan and set aside. Keep warm.
2. Add the remaining olive oil to the pan, along with chopped sage and cinnamon. Cook for about 2-3 minutes, stirring frequently.
3. Return the butternut squash noodles to the pan and toss to coat in sage-cinnamon mixture. Remove the pan from the heat and season with salt and black pepper as desired.
4. Serve immediately with your favorite entrée or as a light main course.

Nutrition Information Per Serving*

Calories: 145

Protein: 1.3 g

Carbohydrates: 15.3 g

Dietary Fiber: 3.2 g

Total Sugars: 2.7 g

Fat: 10.3 g (1.4 g saturated)

* Nutritional information is provided for educational purposes only. [14]

MEDITERRANEAN ROASTED VEGETABLES

This recipe is great for using up extra vegetables from the garden or leftovers so they don't go to waste. Any hearty vegetables (eggplant, carrots, parsnips, and others) can be used in place of the vegetables in the ingredients list below.

Tip

Italian seasoning can be used in place of the Herbs de Provence if desired, this will alter the flavor, but the result will still be delicious.

Prep time: 15 minutes
Cook time: 40-45 minutes
Serves: 4-6

Ingredients
1 pound bag mini sweet peppers, cut in half and seeded
1 pound portobello mushroom caps, sliced
1 large red onion, sliced
1 pound Brussels sprouts, cut off ends and slice in half
2 teaspoons garlic powder
2 teaspoons Herbs de Provence or Italian seasoning
2 tablespoons extra virgin olive oil
2 tablespoons balsamic vinegar
Sea salt and black pepper

Directions

1. Preheat oven to 425 °F and line a large, rimmed baking sheet with parchment paper. Set aside.
2. Add the peppers, portobello mushrooms, onion, and Brussels sprouts to a large mixing bowl. Add the Herbs de Provence, garlic powder, balsamic vinegar, and olive oil. Toss gently to mix. Sprinkle with sea salt and pepper as needed.
3. Arrange the seasoned vegetables on the prepared baking sheet in a single layer. Leave enough space so they aren't overcrowded. Use two large baking sheets, if necessary.
4. Place the sheet pan in preheated oven and roast for 40-45 minutes or until the vegetables are tender and develop a nice caramelized color. Stir halfway through. Remove from the oven and serve immediately. Enjoy!

Nutrition Information Per Serving*

Calories: 135
Protein: 6.1 g
Carbohydrates: 18.3 g
Dietary Fiber: 5.8 g
Total Sugars: 6.4 g
Fat: 6.2 g (1 g saturated)

* Nutritional information is provided for educational purposes only. [14]

Roasted Rosemary Potatoes

These delicious roasted potatoes are colorful and very easy to make. The combination of fresh rosemary paired with garlic and sautéed onions makes them a mouth pleaser. They are the perfect side for most meals.

Prep time: 10 minutes
Cook time: 25-30 minutes
Serves: 4

Ingredients

1 pound tricolored fingerling potatoes, washed, cut in half
2 tablespoons extra virgin olive oil
3 tablespoons fresh rosemary leaves, minced
3 cloves fresh garlic, minced
1 tablespoon coconut oil
2 large white onions, cut into thin strips
Salt and black pepper

Directions

1. Preheat oven to 425 °F.
2. Place a sheet of parchment paper on a rimmed, large baking sheet pan. Set aside.
3. In a large bowl, add potatoes, rosemary leaves, garlic, and olive oil. Toss the ingredients to combine and season with salt and black pepper, as desired.
4. Place the potatoes onto the baking sheet and arrange them in a single layer without overcrowding. Place the pan in the preheated oven and roast for about 15 minutes. Then, turn the potatoes over to brown evenly. Roast the potatoes for about 10-15 minutes more, or until they tender.

5. While the potatoes are cooking, melt coconut oil in a large skillet over medium heat. Add sliced onion and sauté. Stir the onions occasionally, until they turn a deep brown color, approximately 10-15 minutes. Remove from heat and sprinkle with salt and pepper as desired.
6. Remove the pan of potatoes from the oven. Place the potatoes into a serving bowl. Add the onions, mix and serve.

Nutrition Information Per Serving*

Calories: 165

Protein: 1.8 g

Carbohydrates: 13 g

Dietary Fiber: 2.3 g

Total Sugars: 3.2 g

Fat: 12.6 g (4.6 g saturated)

* Nutritional information is provided for educational purposes only. [14]

Tuscan White Beans with Sage

In general, Tuscan cooking is neither fussy nor complicated. It does not depend on costly ingredients, thick sauces, or detailed appearance to stand out. Instead, Tuscan recipes use high-quality local ingredients combined in delicious and simple ways.

This recipe is a good example of a typical Tuscan dish. Humble white beans are infused with garlic flavors, fresh herbs, and spices. Then they are topped off with a drizzle of high-quality extra virgin olive oil for which Tuscany is known.

Healthy Vegan Cooking

I recommend that you make more beans than you need. That way you can always use them in soups, stews, salads, or any recipe that calls for beans.

Tip
Here's a time-saving alternative to soaking the beans overnight, when you are pressed for time. Add the beans to a large pot. Cover them with 3" of cold water. Bring the water to a rapid boil on high heat for one minute, then turn off the heat. Cover and let the pot sit for at least one hour and then drain off the water.

Prep time: 10 minutes + soaking time
Cook time: 1½ - 2 hours
Yields: 6½ - 7 cups

Ingredients
3 cups dried white beans (cannellini is recommended), rinsed
2 tablespoons olive oil
6-8 cloves garlic, peeled and smashed
2 bay leaves
10-12 large fresh sage leaves
2 large sprigs fresh thyme
2 large sprigs fresh rosemary
2 teaspoons sea salt
15-20 whole black peppercorns
2 tablespoons high-quality extra virgin olive oil
Sea salt and black pepper

Directions
1. Add rinsed white beans to a large bowl and add cold water to cover. Put a lid on the bowl and leave the beans to soak for at about 8 hours or overnight.

2. Drain and rinse beans and transfer them to a large stockpot or Dutch oven. Cover with 2-3 inches of cold water. Add olive oil, garlic, bay leaves, fresh herbs, sea salt, and black peppercorns. Bring to a low boil for one minute over medium-high heat, then reduce the heat to medium-low. Remove any foam that gathers on the surface while boiling.
3. Cover and simmer, stir occasionally, for 1 to 1½ hours or until beans are tender. Remove the pot from the heat and let cool with the liquid for about 15-20 minutes.

Note: The cooking time depends on the size and age of the beans. Beans that are fresh and smaller will take less time to cook. Check for doneness after about 45 minutes and adjust the cooking time accordingly. The beans should be soft, but not mushy.

4. Carefully drain the beans, reserving some of the liquid to use in soups or stews, if desired. Remove and any solids that resulted from cooking. Then transfer the beans to a serving container. Add salt and pepper, as desired. Add a small amount of olive oil and mix. Serve and enjoy!

Nutrition Information Per Serving*
Calories: 219
Protein: 8.6 g
Carbohydrates: 24.4 g
Dietary Fiber: 11.6 g
Total Sugars: 1 g
Fat: 10 g (1.6 g saturated)
* Nutritional information is provided for educational purposes only. [14]

CRISPY KALE CHIPS

Here is a healthy and low carb alternative to fried potato chips. These crispy and delicious kale chips are easy to make, but there are several things to be aware of before you begin to prepare them.

First, it is important to find the appropriate combination of oven temperature and cooking time. These chips tend to burn very quickly, so you will want to watch them closely. Especially if it is your first time making them. Here, crispy chips were yielded at 325 °F for only 6-7 minutes. However, your oven may be different, so you will need to watch it closely to see what works best for you to avoid soggy or overly bitter and brown chips.

Next, make sure that the kale is completely dry before baking. If there is any remaining moisture, it will cause steam to form and the chips will be soggy. Also, only a very small amount of olive oil is needed to very lightly coat each kale leaf.

Lastly, you can experiment with different combinations of seasonings if you desire. While sea salt is good by itself, other seasonings like smoked paprika, garlic powder, and ground cumin add more flavor.

Prep time: 10 minutes
Cook time: 6-8 minutes
Serves: 4

Ingredients
2 large bunches kale (about 16-18 ounces)
1½ - 2 tablespoons extra virgin olive oil
1 tablespoon smoked paprika
2 teaspoons garlic powder

2 teaspoons ground cumin
Sea salt

Directions

1. Preheat oven to 325 °F.
2. Line a large baking sheet with parchment paper. Set aside.
3. Wash the kale leaves and dry them completely. Remove the stems and tear them into bite-size pieces before adding them to a large mixing bowl. Lightly drizzle a little olive oil. Then toss to combine and rub each leaf with your fingers to make sure it is evenly coated in oil.
4. On top of the oil-coated kale, sprinkle the garlic powder, cumin, and smoked paprika. Season with sea salt, as desired. Toss the kale until seasonings are evenly combined.
5. Arrange the seasoned kale leaves on the prepared baking sheet in a single layer. Leave enough space to prevent overcrowding. Work in batches, if necessary.
6. Place baking sheet in preheated oven and bake for 5-6 minutes before rotating the pan. Bake for another 1-2 minutes. Do not overcook. Remove the chips from the oven when they are still mostly green, with only a tiny bit of brown.
7. Let chips set for 2-3 minutes to crisp up a bit more before serving. Enjoy!

Nutrition Information Per Serving*

Calories: 126
Protein: 3.9 g
Carbohydrates: 13.8 g
Dietary Fiber: 2.5 g
Total Sugars: 0.5 g

Fat: 7.2 g (1 g saturated)

*Nutritional information is provided for educational purposes only. [14]

SPICY SWEET POTATO WEDGES WITH SAVORY COCONUT YOGURT DIP

These delicious crispy sweet potato wedges are a great healthy alternative to deep-fried potatoes and other unhealthy snacks. The refreshing savory coconut yogurt dip goes well with the spicy seasonings used in this recipe. You can enhance the flavor by refrigerating the savory yogurt dip overnight before serving it to allow more time for the flavors to develop.

Prep time: 10 minutes
Cook time: 30 minutes
Serves: 4

Tip
You will get crispier sweet potato wedges if you wait to salt them until they are done roasting.

Ingredients
2 large sweet potatoes, sliced into wedges
2 tablespoons coconut oil, melted
1 teaspoon ground cumin
1 teaspoon curry powder
1 teaspoon smoked paprika
½ teaspoon cayenne pepper
½ teaspoon ground cinnamon
1 cup coconut yogurt
2 teaspoons fresh lemon juice

3 teaspoons fresh dill, minced

3 tablespoons fresh parsley, minced

Sea salt and black pepper

Directions
1. Preheat the oven to 400 °F.
2. Place parchment paper on a large baking sheet with parchment paper. Set aside.
3. In a large bowl, coat the sweet potatoes with the melted coconut oil.
4. In a small bowl, mix the curry powder, smoked paprika, cayenne pepper, cinnamon, and cumin. Sprinkle the mixture on the sweet potato wedges. Combine so that all the wedges are lightly coated.
5. Arrange the sweet potato wedges on the prepared baking sheet in a single layer. For crispier wedges, do not overcrowd.
6. Put the baking sheet into the preheated oven. Roast the sweet potatoes wedges for about 30-35 minutes until they are golden brown and crispy on the outside. Turn each wedge once after 15 minutes to brown both sides.
7. While the wedges are roasting, prepare the savory coconut yogurt dip. In a small bowl, combine the coconut yogurt, dill, parsley, and lemon juice. Season with salt and pepper as desired. Put coconut yogurt dip in the refrigerator to chill.
8. When the sweet potato wedges are done, remove them from the oven. Sprinkle with salt, as desired. Let them cool slightly before serving. Service them with the coconut yogurt dip. Enjoy!

Nutrition Information Per Serving*

Calories: 166

Protein: 2 g
Carbohydrates: 21 g
Dietary Fiber: 4.4 g
Total Sugars: 5 g
Fat: 8.9 g (8 g saturated)

* Nutritional information is provided for educational purposes only. [14] [15]

CHAPTER 14 – MAIN DISHES

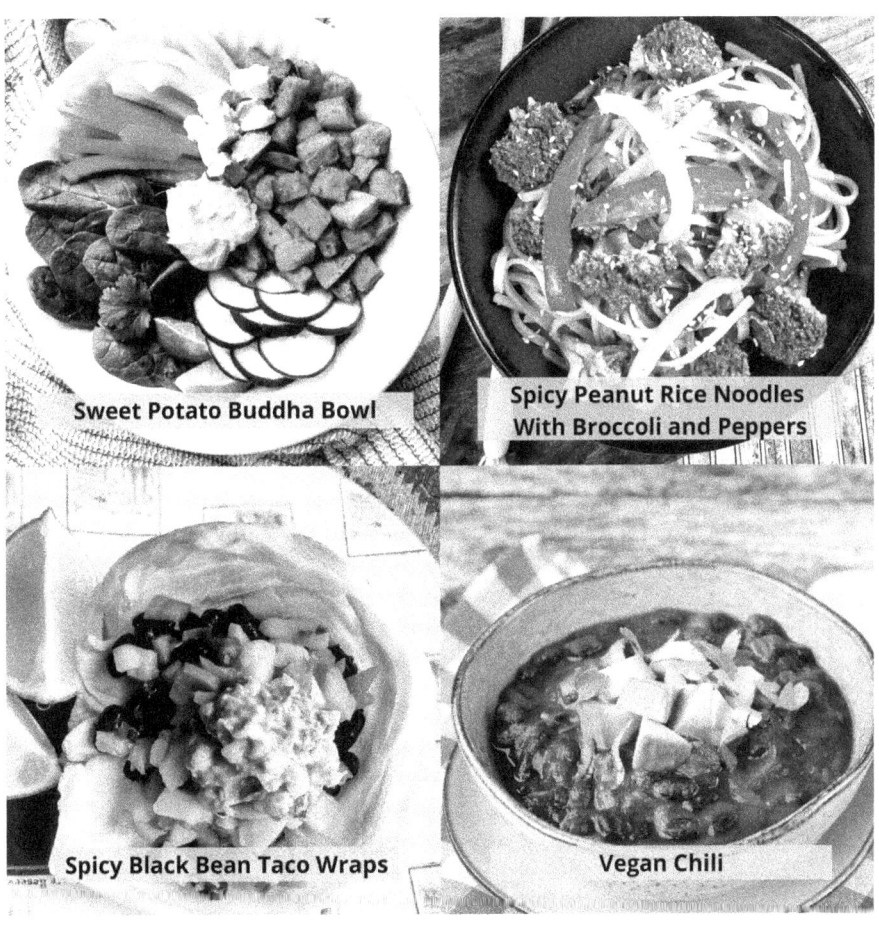

SPICY PEANUT RICE NOODLES WITH BROCCOLI & BELL PEPPERS

Prep time: 15 minutes
Cook time: 10 minutes
Serves: 6

Ingredients

1 14-ounce package rice noodles
3 tablespoons toasted sesame oil, divided
1 pound frozen broccoli florets, divided
8 ounces white mushrooms, cleaned and sliced
1 medium red bell pepper, sliced
1 medium yellow bell pepper, sliced
2 green onions, sliced
1/3 cup soy sauce or coconut aminos
½ cup sugar-free peanut butter
1-2 tablespoons Sriracha sauce

Directions

1. Cook the rice noodles as specified on the package. Set aside.
2. Heat 2 tablespoons sesame oil over medium-high heat in a large frying pan or wok, then add the vegetables and cook. Stir continually, for approximately 5-6 minutes, or until crisp-tender. Remove from heat and set aside.
3. In a medium bowl, whisk the soy sauce, peanut butter, Sriracha, and the remaining sesame oil together until smooth. Add hot water to thin the sauce, if needed.
4. Split the sauce and add half into the vegetables and half into the noodles. Then mix the vegetables and the

noodles together and combine them. Serve immediately. Enjoy!

Nutrition Information Per Serving*
Calories: 400
Protein: 12.2 g
Carbohydrates: 31.2 g
Dietary Fiber: 5.7 g
Total Sugars: 7.3 g
Fat: 26.9 g (5 g saturated)
* Nutritional information is provided for educational purposes only. [14]

Sweet Potato Buddha Bowl with Sriracha Hummus

Prep time: 10 minutes
Cook time: 20 minutes
Serves: 4

Ingredients
2 large sweet potatoes, peeled and cubed
2 tablespoons extra virgin olive oil
1 teaspoon ground cumin
1 teaspoon smoked paprika
6 cups baby spinach
2 red bell peppers, sliced thin
2 yellow bell peppers, sliced thin
2 small cucumbers, thinly sliced
1 cup fresh cilantro, chopped
1 cup plain hummus

2-3 tablespoons sriracha sauce
2 large avocados, cubed
Sea salt and black pepper

Directions
1. Preheat the oven to 400 °F.
2. Place parchment paper on a large baking sheet. Set aside.
3. Add the sweet potato cubes, olive oil, ground cumin, and smoked paprika to a large bowl. Mix until combined. Season with salt and pepper. Next, place the contents on the baking sheet in a single layer, but avoid overcrowding.
4. Place the baking sheet in the preheated oven and roast until the potatoes are fork-tender, around 20 minutes.
5. Divide the sliced peppers, cucumber, spinach, and cilantro into four bowls, while the sweet potato cubes are cooking. Set aside.
6. In a small bowl, use a whisk to combine the hummus and sriracha sauce. Set aside.
7. When the sweet potatoes are finished roasting, remove them from the oven and cool for several minutes. Then divide them between the four Buddha bowls.
8. To serve, top each bowl with diced avocado and a big dollop of sriracha hummus. Enjoy!

Nutrition Information Per Serving*
Calories: 499
Protein: 11.4 g
Carbohydrates: 50.2 g
Dietary Fiber: 15.3 g
Total Sugars: 13 g
Fat: 32.2 g (4.6 g saturated)
* Nutritional information is provided for educational purposes only. [14]

SPICY BLACK BEAN TACO WRAPS WITH GUACAMOLE

These vegan spicy black bean taco wraps are great for a quick meal and only take about 20 minutes to make.

Prep time: 15 minutes
Cook time: 5 minutes
Serves: 4

Ingredients
2 tablespoons extra virgin olive oil
one 15-ounce can black beans, drained and rinsed
2 tablespoons water
1 teaspoon ground cumin
½ teaspoon chili powder
1 teaspoon smoked paprika
¼ teaspoon cayenne pepper
¼ teaspoon dried Mexican oregano
Sea salt and black pepper
Optional: ½ medium red bell pepper, diced

Guacamole Ingredients
2 large ripe avocados, pitted
1 medium tomato, seeded and diced
3 tablespoons fresh lime juice
2 tablespoons fresh cilantro, minced
½ medium jalapeño, finely diced
Sea salt and black pepper

To Serve
Spicy mango salsa*
Lettuce (iceberg, or romaine) leaves for wrapping

Directions

1. In a pan over medium heat, heat the olive oil. Then add the beans, chili powder, cumin, cayenne, smoked paprika, Mexican oregano, and water. Season with salt and pepper. Stir to mix thoroughly.
2. Cook and stir occasionally until the beans are warmed through, and the spices become fragrant, around 4-5 minutes. Remove the pan from the heat.
3. Prepare the guacamole while the beans are cooking. In a small glass bowl, mash the avocado to soften. Then add the tomato, cilantro, jalapeño, and lime juice. Add salt and pepper, as desired. Stir to combine. Set aside.
4. Transfer the warm beans to a bowl and add diced bell pepper, if using. Sprinkle with extra spices, if desired. Serve immediately. Use the large lettuce leaves for wrapping with the fresh guacamole and spicy mango salsa*. Enjoy!

*See chapter 8 for the spicy mango salsa recipe.

Nutrition Information Per Serving*

Calories: 326
Protein: 8.3 g
Carbohydrates: 31.4 g
Dietary Fiber: 12.1 g
Total Sugars: 3.3 g
Fat: 21.2 g (2.9 g saturated)

* Nutritional information is provided for educational purposes only. [14]

VEGGIE BURGERS

Prep Time: 10 minutes
Cook Time: 55 minutes
Serves: 6

Ingredients

10 ounces cauliflower rice
8 ounces mushrooms, finely diced
½ cup onion, finely diced
½ cup celery, finely diced
2 cloves garlic, minced
1 tablespoon olive oil
1 teaspoon tamari sauce
¼ teaspoon paprika, smoked
1 teaspoon parsley, dried
¼ teaspoon cumin, ground
¼ teaspoon garlic powder
½ teaspoon sea salt
1 tablespoon chia seeds
¼ cup golden flax meal

Directions

1. Place the olive oil in a large pan over medium heat before adding the garlic, celery, and onion. Allow the veggies to cook for two to three minutes until they begin to soften. Add in the cauliflower rice and mushrooms, continuing to cook and stir for ten to twelve minutes. You will want to cook this until much of the moisture is cooked out of the vegetables as possible. Remove the pan from the heat.
2. Preheat your oven to the hot temperature of four-hundred degrees Fahrenheit.

3. Add the soy sauce and seasonings to the vegetable burger mixture, combining it well. Add in the chia seeds and flax seeds, combining them until combined. Set the mixture aside and let it cool down for five to ten minutes, which will allow it to thicken.
4. Line a large baking sheet with parchment paper (not a silicone mat). Once the vegetable mixture has cooled down, divide it into four evenly sized patties. The mixture will be sticky but should easily come together. It is best to oil your hands to prevent the mixture from sticking.
5. If your vegetable mixture doesn't stick together well, add one or two more tablespoons of flaxseed meal. Give it a few minutes to absorb before making the patties.
6. Place the pan of burgers into the center of the preheated oven. Bake until they are brown and crispy, about thirty minutes. Then remove the burgers from the oven and allow them to cool for five minutes before serving.

Nutrition Information Per Serving*

Calories: 143

Protein: 6.9 g

Carbohydrates: 12.2 g

Dietary Fiber: 5.6 g

Total Sugars: 3.1 g

Fat: 9.2 g (0.7 g saturated)

* Nutritional information is provided for educational purposes only. [14]

HERB ROASTED VEGGIES

Prep Time: 10 minutes
Cook Time: 35 minutes
Serves: 6

Ingredients
1½ pounds new potatoes, quartered
½ cup baby carrots
1 small onion, cut into wedges
¼ cup olive oil
3 tablespoons lemon juice
3 cloves garlic, minced
1 tablespoon chopped fresh rosemary
1 tablespoon dried oregano
½ small eggplant, quartered and cut into 1/2-inch strips
1 red bell pepper, cut into strips, 1/2-inch wide
Salt and pepper

Directions
1. Preheat the oven to 450 °F.
2. In a 13x9 inch baking pan, ungreased, add the potatoes, onion, and carrots.
3. In a small bowl, add the olive oil, lemon juice, rosemary, garlic, oregano, and salt and pepper, as desired. Stir to mix. Next, pour the mixture over the vegetables in the baking pan.
4. Place the baking pan with the vegetables in the oven and roast for 20 minutes.
5. Remove the baking pan from the oven and add the eggplant and bell pepper. Stir to combine. Place the baking pan back into the oven.

6. Roast for 13 to 15 more minutes or until the vegetables are tender and brown on the edges. Serve hot.

Nutrition Information Per Serving*
Calories: 182
Protein: 2.9 g
Carbohydrates: 24.8 g
Dietary Fiber: 5.5 g
Total Sugars: 4.6 g
Fat: 8.9 g (1.4 g saturated)
* Nutritional information is provided for educational purposes only. [14]

VEGAN CHILI

Prep Time: 20 minutes
Cook Time: 40 minutes
Serves: 4-6

Ingredients
2 tablespoons extra-virgin olive oil
1 medium red onion, chopped
1 large red bell pepper, chopped
2 medium carrots, chopped
2 celery ribs, chopped
½ teaspoon salt, divided
4 cloves garlic, pressed or minced
2 tablespoons chili powder
2 teaspoons ground cumin
1½ teaspoons smoked paprika
1 teaspoon dried oregano

one 28-ounce can of diced tomatoes, with juice

two 15-ounce cans of black beans, rinsed and drained

one 15-ounce can of pinto beans, rinsed and drained

2 cups vegetable broth or water

1 bay leaf

2 teaspoons fresh cilantro, chopped, plus enough for garnish

1-2 teaspoons red wine vinegar or lime juice

Garnishes: sliced avocado, tortilla chips, vegan sour cream, chopped cilantro

Directions

1. In a large pot (heavy bottom), heat the olive oil over medium heat. Next add onion, bell pepper, carrots, celery, and ¼ teaspoon of salt. Mix and stir occasionally until the onion is translucent and vegetables are tender, about 7-10 minutes.
2. Then add the chili powder, cumin, garlic, paprika, and oregano. Cook and stir frequently for about 1 minute.
3. Next add the diced tomatoes, black beans, pinto beans, vegetable broth, and bay leaf. Mix and allow it to simmer. Then allow to cook at a gentle simmer (adjust heat as needed) for 30 minutes and stir occasionally.
4. Take 1½ cups of the chili with liquid, place in a blender, and blend until smooth. Then return it back into the pot.
5. Now add the cilantro and stir to mix. Then add the desired amount of vinegar for your taste and mix. Add the remaining ¼ teaspoon of salt to the pot.
6. Place the chili into bowls and add your desired garnishes.
7. Store the remaining chili in the refrigerator for about 4 days or longer if frozen.

Nutrition Information Per Serving*

Calories: 486

Protein: 25.9 g
Carbohydrates: 81 g
Dietary Fiber: 28.5 g
Total Sugars: 13.8 g
Fat: 9 g (1 g saturated)
* Nutritional information is provided for educational purposes only. [14]

VEGAN PITA PIZZAS

Prep Time: 10 minutes
Cook Time: 20 minutes
Serves: 6 pizzas

Ingredients
6 whole-wheat pitas

Tomato Sauce Ingredients
2 large tomatoes, diced
4 sun-dried tomatoes
2 tablespoons tomato puree
5 teaspoons maple syrup
1 tablespoon apple cider vinegar
2 cloves garlic
1 tablespoon dried oregano
1 handful of fresh basil
5 teaspoons dried thyme
Salt and pepper

Toppings
1 cup olives, halved

½ cup smoked tofu, diced
10 pickled peperoncino, sliced
½ zucchini, thinly sliced
3 tablespoons vegan parmesan
fresh basil

Directions
1. Preheat oven at 400 °F.
2. First, prepare the toppings. Dice the tofu and cut the olives in half. Slice the zucchini and the peperoncino.
3. Dice the tomatoes. Place the tomato sauce ingredients into a blender. Blend until smooth.
4. Place the pitas on a baking sheet. Spread the tomato sauce evenly on each pita. Add the other toppings, except the Parmesan and fresh basil.
5. Place the baking sheet with the pitas in the oven and bake for 15-20 minutes.
6. Top with Parmesan and basil and serve.

Nutrition Information Per Serving*
Calories: 170
Protein: 6.8 g
Carbohydrates: 29 g
Dietary Fiber: 5 g
Total Sugars: 5.4 g
Fat: 4.7 g (0.7 g saturated)
* Nutritional information is provided for educational purposes only. [14]

CHAPTER 15 – DESSERTS

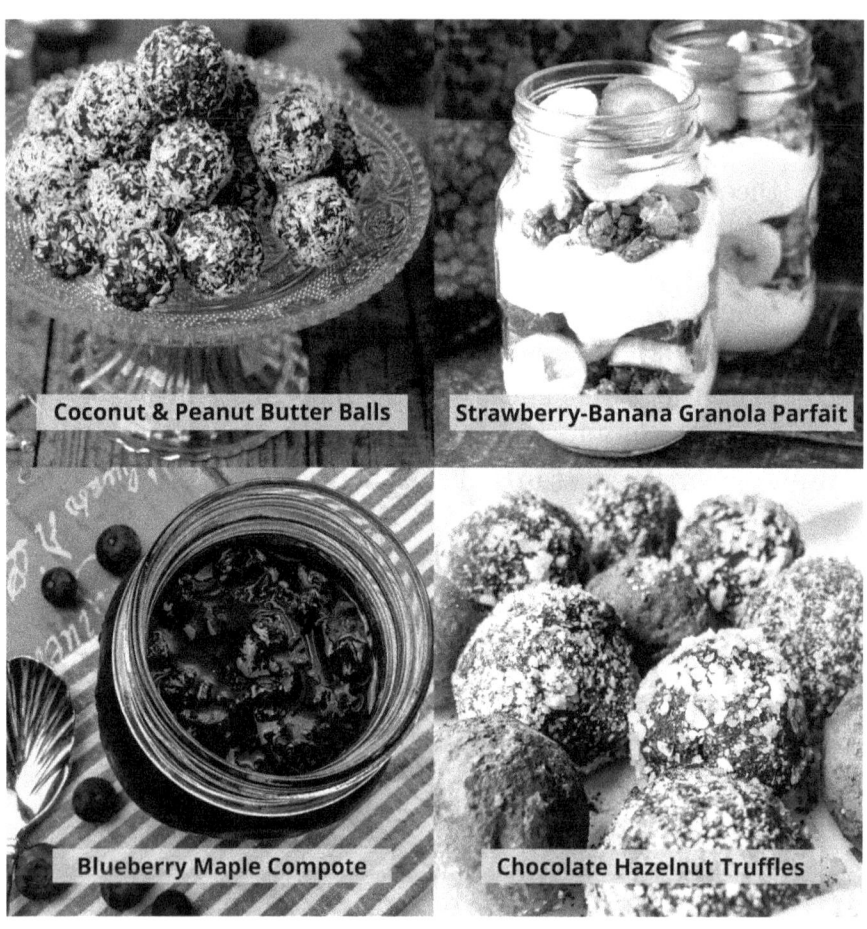

INSTANT POT BLUEBERRY MAPLE COMPOTE

Classic compote recipes typically include large amounts of white sugar. However, this recipe uses more real maple syrup for a taste of sweetness. While this recipe uses fresh blueberries, lemon juice, and cinnamon, feel free to add any combination of fresh berries, citrus juice, and seasonings to create your own tasty flavor variations.

Prep time: 5 minutes
Cook time: 13 minutes + time to come to pressure
Makes 3 cups
Serves: 4

Ingredients
3 cups fresh or frozen blueberries

¼ cup real maple syrup

2 tablespoons fresh lemon juice

1 teaspoon vanilla extract

1 teaspoon ground cinnamon

¼ teaspoon salt

Directions
1. Add all ingredients to the Instant Pot container and stir to combine. Add the lid and lock it into position.
2. Set the Instant Pot's pressure valve to the "Sealing" position and then press the "Manual" button. Adjust the setting to high and select 3 minutes for the cooking time. The Instant Pot will begin building pressure after a short amount of time.
3. When the cooking time has finished, turn the Instant Pot off to prevent scorching. Wait for about 10 minutes to allow most of the pressure to release naturally. Now

move the valve to the "Venting" position to release any remaining pressure.

4. Optional: If you want to thicken the compote, set the "Sauté" function to cook on high heat. Stir constantly until the excess liquid is reduced. Turn the Instant Pot off and immediately remove the container from the unit to cool.
5. Serve immediately or transfer to an airtight container and store in the refrigerator for 7 to 10 days. Enjoy!

Nutrition Information Per Serving*
Calories: 120
Protein: 1 g
Carbohydrates: 29.7 g
Dietary Fiber: 3 g
Total Sugars: 22.8 g
Fat: 0.5 g (0.1 g saturated)
* Nutritional information is provided for educational purposes only. [14]

CHOCOLATE HAZELNUT TRUFFLES

These decadent chocolate hazelnut truffles are a delicious snack that is sure to satisfy your sweet tooth. The combination of dates and a small amount of maple syrup provide enough sweetness. And the best part is no refined sugar is used. And, the cocoa powder adds a nice chocolate taste while keeping it vegan-friendly.

Prep time: 25 minutes
Cook time: n/a
Yield: 15-18 truffles

Ingredients

½ cup raw hazelnuts

12 Medjool dates, pitted

2 tablespoons cocoa powder, unsweetened

2 tablespoons coconut flour

1 tablespoon coconut oil, melted

1½ tablespoons pure maple syrup

1 teaspoon pure vanilla extract

¼ teaspoon coarse salt

Optional Coatings

¼ cup hazelnuts or almonds, ground

¼ cup coconut flakes, finely shredded

2 tablespoons unsweetened cocoa powder + ¼ teaspoon each cayenne pepper and coarse salt

Directions

1. Place the pitted dates in a small bowl filled with warm water and soak for 10-15 minutes.
2. Line a rimmed baking sheet with wax paper and set aside. If you use the optional coating, mix the optional coating ingredients in a shallow bowl and set aside.
3. Add hazelnuts to a food processor and process until finely ground.
4. Remove the softened dates from the bowl and drain off any excess water. Add the dates and cocoa powder to the food processor and blend until smooth, approximately 3-4 minutes. Scrape the sides, as necessary, to ensure that the mixture is thoroughly combined.

    Tip: You can add a couple of drops of water at a time, as needed, to smooth out the mixture. However, care should be taken to not add too much water.

5. Add the salt, coconut flour, maple syrup, coconut oil, and vanilla extract to the mixture in the food processor and mix until combined.
6. Remove the dough from the food processor and divide it into 15-18 equal-sized portions. Roll each portion of dough into a ball. Then roll it in the optional coating mixture if used.
7. Next, place the balls on the prepared baking tray. Refrigerate to chill for several minutes before serving. Enjoy!

Nutrition Information Per Serving (1 truffle)*
Calories: 145
Protein: 1.5 g
Carbohydrates: 30.5 g
Dietary Fiber: 3.5 g
Total Sugars: 23.1 g
Fat: 2.8 g (1.4 g saturated)
* Nutritional information is provided for educational purposes only. [14]

BLUEBERRY & CASHEW CHEESECAKE

Prep time: 20 minutes + chill time
Cook time: n/a
Serves: 8

Crust Ingredients
1 teaspoon cinnamon
2 tablespoons desiccated coconut
2 tablespoons ground flax seeds

Filling Ingredients
1 cup of soaked cashews
4 ounces vegan cream cheese
1 tablespoon lemon juice
2 tablespoons coconut oil
½ cup blueberries (raw or frozen)
1 teaspoons vanilla extract
2 tablespoons agave or maple syrup

Directions
1. Soak the cashews in a bowl of warm water for a minimum of 3 hours.
2. Mix all the crust ingredients and flatten them into a regular pie dish.
3. Combine all the filling ingredients in a high powered blender until smooth.
4. Empty the filling into a container and chill until firm.
5. Optional: top with blueberries

Nutrition Information Per Serving*
Calories: 177
Protein: 2.4 g
Carbohydrates: 5 g
Dietary Fiber: 1.2 g
Total Sugars: 1.5 g
Fat: 16.3 g (9 g saturated)

* Nutritional information is provided for educational purposes only [14]

BLUEBERRY & PECAN CRUMBLE

Prep time: 10 minutes
Cook time: 30 minutes
Serves: 6

Ingredients
3 tablespoons chia seeds
1 tablespoon lemon juice
14 ounces blueberries
1 ½ teaspoon stevia powder
2 cups blanched almond flour
2 tablespoons cinnamon
¼ cup chopped pecans
5 tablespoons coconut oil

Directions
1. Preheat the oven to 400 °F.
2. Prepare a cast-iron skillet. Combine the berries, stevia, chia seeds, and lemon juice and add to the skillet.
3. Mix the rest of the ingredients in a bowl and spread over the skillet of berries.
4. Add the skillet to the hot oven and bake for 30 minutes.
5. Remove from the oven and serve.

Nutrition Information Per Serving*
Calories: 235
Protein: 4.2 g
Carbohydrates: 16.8 g
Dietary Fiber: 6.5 g
Total Sugars: 6.9 g
Fat: 19.4 g (10.4 g saturated)

* Nutritional information is provided for educational purposes only. [14]

CINNAMON & PUMPKIN FUDGE

Prep time: 10 minutes + 2 hours in the refrigerator
Cook time: n/a
Servings: 24

Ingredients
¼ teaspoon ground nutmeg

1 teaspoon ground cinnamon

1 cup pumpkin puree

1 ¾ cups warmed/melted coconut butter

1 tablespoon coconut oil

Directions
1. Combine the ingredients (coconut butter, spices, and pumpkin). Whisk in the coconut oil.
2. Spread the mixture over a foil-lined baking dish and cover with wax paper. Press out the fudge until even. Discard the paper and place it in the refrigerator for 2 hours.
3. Cut into squares.

Nutrition Information Per Serving*
Calories: 127

Protein: 1.2 g

Carbohydrates: 5.2 g

Dietary Fiber: 3.6 g

Total Sugars: 1.4 g

Fat: 11.9 g (10.7 g saturated)

* Nutritional information is provided for educational purposes only. [14]

Coconut Maple Fudge

Prep time: 7 minutes + refrigerator time
Cook time: n/a
Servings: 18

Ingredients
½ cup Coconut oil

½ cup Coconut butter

1 teaspoon maple extract

½ cup coconut, shredded, unsweetened, toasted

½ teaspoon liquid stevia coconut sweet drops

Directions
1. Add a layer of parchment paper to a baking sheet.
2. Melt the coconut butter and oil in a pan (low heat). Combine remaining ingredients except for the shredded coconut.
3. Sprinkle the shredded coconut on the prepared baking sheet. Pour the mixture over the coconut.
4. Place in the refrigerator to firm up. Then, cut into 18 pieces and enjoy!

Nutrition Information Per Serving*
Calories: 66
Protein: 0.6 g
Carbohydrates: 2.3 g
Dietary Fiber: 1.7 g
Total Sugars: 0.6 g
Fat: 6.4 g (5.8 g saturated)
* Nutritional information is provided for educational purposes only. [14]

Coconut & Peanut Butter Balls

Prep time: 1.25 hour + refrigerator time (overnight)
Cook time: n/a
Servings: 15

Ingredients
3 teaspoons unsweetened cocoa powder
3 tablespoons creamy peanut butter, vegan-friendly
2 teaspoons almond flour
4 drops liquid stevia
½ cup coconut flakes

Directions
1. Combine the peanut butter, cocoa, stevia, and flour in a bowl. Place the bowl in the freezer for 1 hour.
2. Using a small spoon, prepare the servings, and drop into the coconut flakes.
3. Roll them around and reshape if needed.
4. Refrigerate until firm.

Nutrition Information Per Serving*
Calories: 31
Protein: 1 g
Carbohydrates: 1.3 g
Dietary Fiber: 0.6g
Total Sugars: 0.5 g
Fat: 2.7 g (1.2 g saturated)
* Nutritional information is provided for educational purposes only. [14]

Chia Raspberry Pudding

Prep time: 7 minutes + refrigerator time (overnight)
Cook time: n/a
Servings: 4

Ingredients

1 cup coconut milk
½ cup water
1 cup fresh raspberries
½ cup whole chia seeds
1 teaspoon vanilla powder

Directions

1. Mix the raspberries, milk, and water in a blender until smooth.
2. Pour mixture into a bowl and fold in the chia seeds and vanilla.
3. Chill the pudding overnight in the refrigerator for best results.

Nutrition Information Per Serving*

Calories: 181
Protein: 1.7 g
Carbohydrates: 7.3 g
Dietary Fiber: 3.3 g
Total Sugars: 3.6 g
Fat: 14.5 g (12.7 g saturated)

* Nutritional information is provided for educational purposes only. [14]

PUMPKIN AND PEANUT BUTTER PUDDING

Prep time: 5 minutes + refrigerator time (overnight)
Cook time: n/a
Servings: 2

Ingredients
½ cup pumpkin puree

½ cup peanut butter

2 tablespoons chia seeds

1 cup coconut milk

Directions
1. Place the ingredients into a blender.
2. Blend the ingredients on high for 1 minute and pour the mixture into a mason jar.
3. Refrigerate to chill, preferably overnight.

Nutrition Information Per Serving*
Calories: 725

Protein: 22.4 g

Carbohydrates: 28.1 g

Dietary Fiber: 12.2 g

Total Sugars: 11 g

Fat: 66.1 g (32.6 g saturated)

* Nutritional information is provided for educational purposes only. [14]

STRAWBERRY BANANA GRANOLA PARFAITS

Prep time: 10 minutes
Cook time: 20 minutes
Servings: 4

Ingredients
6 large dates, pitted
3 tablespoons almond butter
3 tablespoons maple syrup
2 tablespoons coconut oil, melted
1 teaspoon real vanilla extract
1 cup rolled oats
½ teaspoon ground cinnamon
¼ teaspoon salt
¼ cup raw almonds, roughly chopped
2 tablespoons sunflower seeds
2 cups coconut yogurt
2 large bananas, sliced
1 cup fresh strawberries, sliced

Directions
1. Preheat oven to 350 °F.
2. Line an 8x8 inch baking pan with parchment paper, leaving overlap on the sides.
3. Add the pitted dates, almond butter, maple syrup, coconut oil, and vanilla extract into a high-powered blender or food processor. Blend the ingredients until the mixture is creamy and smooth.
4. Transfer the mixture to a large mixing bowl. Then add the oats, cinnamon, salt, almonds, and sunflower seeds.

Mix until thoroughly combined and the oats and nuts are adequately coated.

5. Transfer the granola mixture to the prepared baking pan and arrange it into an even layer. Place the pan in the preheated oven and bake until lightly golden brown and toasted on top, approximately 20 minutes.
6. Remove the baking pan from the oven and allow it cool to room temperature. Note that the granola will crumble when removed from the pan.
7. To serve, alternate layers of coconut yogurt, granola, sliced bananas, and fresh strawberries in 4 parfait dishes. Enjoy!

Nutrition Information Per Serving*

Calories: 692

Protein: 11.8 g

Carbohydrates: 117.4 g

Dietary Fiber: 8.3 g

Total Sugars: 82.2.6 g

Fat: 22 g (8.8 g saturated)

* Nutritional information is provided for educational purposes only. [14]

FROM THE AUTHOR

First of all, thank you for purchasing this book *"Healthy Vegan Cooking."* While you could have picked any number of books to read, you picked this one, and for that, I am very grateful.

I hope that it added value to your everyday life. If so, it would be nice if you would share this book with your family and friends by posting to Twitter, Facebook, and other social media.

Also, if you enjoyed this book and found it beneficial, I'd like to hear from you. I hope that you could take some time to post a review. Your feedback and support will greatly help me improve my writing for future projects and make this book even better.

If you would like to leave a review, all you have to do is to click on the following link for the *"Healthy Vegan Cooking"* book page and select the store of your choice; https://books2read.com/u/mZKDJe.

Finally, if you'd like to get notifications of new book releases, special offers, and other related content, please join my email list at https://www.restoreyourhealthsecrets.com and get your free copy of *"Restore Your Health With Whole Food."*

REFERENCES

1. Moore, J. X., Chaudhary, N., & Akinyemiju, T. (2017). Peer reviewed: Metabolic syndrome prevalence by race/ethnicity and sex in the United States, National Health and Nutrition Examination Survey, 1988–2012. Preventing chronic disease, 14.

2. Grant, J. D. (2017). Time for change: Benefits of a plant-based diet. Canadian Family Physician, 63(10), 744-746

3. Donovan, U. M., & Gibson, R. S. (1996). Dietary intakes of adolescent females consuming vegetarian, semi-vegetarian, and omnivorous diets. Journal of Adolescent Health, 18(4), 292-300.

4. Conrad, Z., Karlsen, M., Chui, K., & Jahns, L. (2017). Diet quality on meatless days: National health and nutrition examination survey (NHANES), 2007–2012. Public health nutrition, 20(9), 1564-1573.

5. Sharifi, N., & Majlessi, F. (2016). Self-empowerment of female students in prevention of osteoporosis. Global Journal of Health Science, 9(2), 7.

6. Kune, S., Kune, G.A. and Watson, L.F., 2017. Case-control study of dietary etiological factors: The Melbourne colorectal cancer study. Nutrition and cancer, 9(1), pp.21-42.

7. Radnitz, C., Beezhold, B., & DiMatteo, J. (2015). Investigation of lifestyle choices of individuals following a vegan diet for health and ethical reasons. Appetite, 90, 31-36.

8. Cohen, E., Cragg, M., deFonseka, J., Hite, A., Rosenberg, M., & Zhou, B. (2015). Statistical review of US macronutrient consumption

data, 1965–2011: Americans have been following dietary guidelines, coincident with the rise in obesity. Nutrition, 31(5), 727-732.

9. Curtiss, C. F., & Craig, J. A. (2017). Economical production of beef. Bulletin, 4(48), 1.

10. Walters, D. E. (2019). Animal Agriculture Liability for Climatic Nuisance: A Path Forward for Climate Change Litigation. Colum. J. Envtl. L., 44, 299.

11. Smith, Jeffrey M. "Health Risks." *Institute for Responsible Technology*, 2015. Web Retrieved January 5, 2020, from https://responsibletechnology.org/gmo-education/health-risks/.

12. "What Is Gelatin Made of?" *PETA*, July 7 2010, Web Retrieved January 5, 2020, from https://www.peta.org/about-peta/faq/what-is-gelatin-made-of/.

13. "Recipe Analyzer." *HappyForks*, happyforks.com/analyzer. Web Retrieved December 17, 2019, from https://happyforks.com/analyzer.

14. Verywell, Team. "Try Our Recipe Nutrition Calculator." *Verywell Fit*, Verywell Fit, February 5, 2018. Web Retrieved December 17, 2019, from https://www.verywellfit.com/recipe-nutrition-analyzer-4157076.

15. White, Dana Angelo, and Atc. "All About Coconut Yogurt." *Verywell Fit*, Verywell Fit, January 31, 2020. Web Retrieved December 17, 2019, from https://www.verywellfit.com/all-about-coconut-yogurt-4165922.

16. "What Is Gelatin Made of?" *PETA*, July 7, 2010. Web Retrieved December 18, 2019, from https://www.kidney.org/atoz/content/what-plant-based-diet-and-it-good-kidney-disease.

17. "Study: Plant-Based Diet Reduces Diabetic Neuropathy Pain." *Fanatic Cook*, August 12, 2014. Web Retrieved December 18, 2019, from https://fanaticcook.com/2014/08/12/study-plant-based-diet-reduces-diabetic-neuropathy-pain/.

18. Katherine Zeratsky, R.D. "Does Soy Really Affect Breast Cancer Risk?" *Mayo Clinic*, Mayo Foundation for Medical Education and Research. Web Retrieved December 18, 2019, from https://www.mayoclinic.org/healthy-lifestyle/nutrition-and-healthy-eating/expert-answers/soy-breast-cancer-risk/faq-20120377.

19. "Animal Protein and Cancer Risk." *UCSF Osher Center for Integrative Medicine*. Web Retrieved December 18, 2019, from https://osher.ucsf.edu/patient-care/integrative-medicine-resources/cancer-and-nutrition/faq/animal-protein-cancer-risk.

20. "History." *The Vegan Society*. Web Retrieved December 18, 2019, from https://www.vegansociety.com/about-us/history.

21. "The Vegan Society." *Wikipedia*, Wikimedia Foundation. Web Retrieved December 18, 2019, from https://en.wikipedia.org/wiki/The_Vegan_Society.

22. Forgrieve, Janet. "The Growing Acceptance Of Veganism." Forbes, November 2, 2018. Web Retrieved December 18, 2019, from https://www.forbes.com/sites/janetforgrieve/2018/11/02/picturing-a-kindler-gentler-world-vegan-month/.

23. Madigan, Mariah, and Elisa Karhu. "The Role of Plant-Based Nutrition in Cancer Prevention." *Journal of Unexplored Medical Data*, November 8, 2018. Web Retrieved December 18, 2019, from https://jumdjournal.net/article/view/2892.

24. Mastroianni, Brian. "Plant-Based Diets Can Reduce Risk of Death from Heart Disease by 10%." *Healthline*, March 19, 2019. Web Retrieved December 18, 2019, from https://www.healthline.com/health-news/incorporating-high-quality-plant-based-foods-to-diet-decreases-risk-of-deaths-from-heart-disease.

25. Young, Micaela. "This Is How Much Protein You Need to Eat Every Day." *EatingWell*. Web Retrieved December 25, 2019, from http://www.eatingwell.com/article/290496/this-is-how-much-protein-you-need-to-eat-every-day/.

26. Sugg, Hayley. "The 10 Best Vegan Protein Sources." *EatingWell*. Web Retrieved December 25, 2019, from http://www.eatingwell.com/article/291111/the-10-best-vegan-protein-sources/.

27. Villines, Zawn. "15 Best Plant-Based Protein Foods." *Medical News Today*, MediLexicon International, April 12, 2018. Web Retrieved December 25, 2019, https://www.medicalnewstoday.com/articles/321474.php.

28. Firman, Tehrene. "How To Get Enough Calcium When You're Vegan or Dairy-Free." *Well+Good*, October 4, 2018. Web Retrieved December 27, 2019, from https://www.wellandgood.com/good-food/vegan-sources-of-calcium/.

29. Mangels, Reed. "Calcium in the Vegan Diet." *The Vegan Resource Group*. Web Retrieved December 27, 2019, from https://www.vrg.org/nutrition/calcium.php.

30. "Vegetarian Calcium Food Sources." *Oldways*. Web Retrieved December 27, 2019, from https://oldwayspt.org/programs/oldways-vegetarian-network/oldways-vegetarian-network-resources/vegetarian-calcium-food.

31. Barhum, Lana. "Calcium-Rich Foods That Vegans Can Eat." *Medical News Today.* Web Retrieved December 27, 2019, from https://www.medicalnewstoday.com/articles/322585.php#non-dairy-sources-of-calcium.

32. "People for the Ethical Treatment of Animals (PETA)." *PETA.* Web Retrieved January 21, 2020, from https://www.peta.org.

33. Brown, Mary Jane. "8 Health Benefits of Probiotics." *Healthline*, August 23, 2016. Web Retrieved January 21, 2020, from https://www.healthline.com/nutrition/8-health-benefits-of-probiotics.

34. Pelz, Dr. Mindy. "Is Your Gut Bacteria Causing You a Mineral Deficiency?", *Dr. Mindy Pelz.* Web Retrieved January 21, 2020, from https://drmindypelz.com/is-your-gut-bacteria-causing-you-a-mineral-deficiency/.

35. Lang, Angela. "Fruits & Vegetables High in Enzymes." *LIVESTRONG.COM.* Web Retrieved January 22, 2020. from https://www.livestrong.com/article/320914-fruits-vegetables-high-in-enzymes/.

36. Raman, Ryan. "12 Healthy Foods High in Antioxidants." *Healthline*, March 12, 2018. Web Retrieved January 22, 2020, from https://www.healthline.com/nutrition/foods-high-in-antioxidants.

37. Rossiter, Brian. "A Quick Guide to a Low-Fat Raw Food Diet, Fruitarian Diet and Fruit Diet." *Fruit-Powered.* Web Retrieved January 22, 2020, from https://www.fruit-powered.com/low-fat-raw-food-diet-fruitarian-diet-fruit-diet/.

38. Ware, Megan. "What Are the Health Benefits of Pumpkins?" *Medical News Today.* Web Retrieved January 22, 2020, from https://www.medicalnewstoday.com/articles/279610.php.

39. Wheeler, Kathryn. "5 Types of Vegan." *Happiful Magazine,* November 1, 2017. Web Retrieved March 19, 2020, from https://happiful.com/5-types-of-vegan/.

40. Hackett, Jolinda. "The Many Different Types of Vegetarian Diets." The Spruce Eats, August 19, 2019. Web Retrieved March 19, 2020, from https://www.thespruceeats.com/types-of-vegetarians-3378611.

About The Author

Thomas Calabris is a health and wellness coach. He has studied anatomy and physiology and many areas of natural health. He has studied and practiced many forms of meditation and Qigong for more than thirty years. He studied meditation, Qigong, and Tai Chi with Grandmaster Robert Krueger. He studied Inner Dan Arts Qigong (meditation, breathing, exercise, and healing) with Grandmaster Tianyou Hao. Thomas is a certified instructor of Inner Dan Arts Qigong. He has also studied Qinway Qigong with Grandmaster Qinyin and Wisdom Healing Qigong with Master Mingtong Gu. He holds a Bachelor of Science Degree in Electrical Engineering and a Master of Science Degree in Biomedical Engineering. He is also a software engineer. He brings a unique perspective of science, tradition, and experience to his teachings. It is his mission to empower people to take charge of their health and wellness through natural and holistic practices like meditation, Qigong, Tai Chi, and healthy eating.

Learn more about the vegan diet at:
https://www.SimpleVeganDiet.com

Learn more about stress relief at:
https://www.EliminateStressNow.com

Learn more about Qigong at:
http://www.InnerVitalityQigong.com

Books By The Author

Relax Your Mind: Simple Meditation Techniques to Relieve Stress and Quiet a Busy Mind

Learn more at: https://www.amazon.com/dp/B07H1PMN62

Relax Your Mind Companion Workbook: A Guide To Learn Meditation Techniques to Relieve Stress and Quiet a Busy Mind

Learn more at: https://www.amazon.com/dp/B07YRWVZSJ

Healing Stress: Effective Solutions for Relieving Stress and Living a Stress-Free Life

Learn more at: https://www.amazon.com/dp/B07KVNXN14

The Color of Relaxation: Adult Coloring Book for Stress Relief and Relaxation

Learn more at: https://www.amazon.com/gp/product/1086248295

Dreams Into Reality: Manifest Your Dreams Into Being Using The Law Of Attraction

Learn more at: https://www.amazon.com/dp/B081NVJ94G

www.ingramcontent.com/pod-product-compliance
Lightning Source LLC
Chambersburg PA
CBHW061325040426
42444CB00011B/2783